Examination Notes in Psychiatry

BASIC SCIENCES

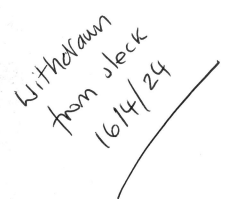
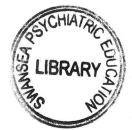
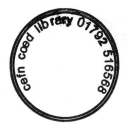

Examination Notes in Psychiatry

BASIC SCIENCES

2nd edition

GIN S. MALHI MBChB BSc(Hons) MRCPsych FRANZCP
School of Psychiatry, University of New South Wales,
Sydney, Australia

SAJ MALHI MBChB MRCPsych
South Kensington and Chelsea Mental Health Centre,
London, UK

Hodder Arnold

A MEMBER OF THE HODDER HEADLINE GROUP
LONDON

First published in Great Britain in 1999 by Butterworth Heinemann
This second edition published in 2006 by
Hodder Arnold, an imprint of Hodder Education and a member of the Hodder Headline Group,
338 Euston Road, London NW1 3BH

http://www.hoddereducation.com

Distributed in the United States of America by
Oxford University Press Inc.,
198 Madison Avenue, New York, NY10016
Oxford is a registered trademark of Oxford University Press

Whilst the advice and information in this book are believed to be true and accurate at the date of
going to press, neither the author[s] nor the publisher can accept any legal responsibility or liability
for any errors or omissions that may be made. In particular (but without limiting the generality of the
preceding disclaimer) every effort has been made to check drug dosages; however it is still possible
that errors have been missed. Furthermore, dosage schedules are constantly being revised and new
side-effects recognized. For these reasons the reader is strongly urged to consult the drug companies'
printed instructions before administering any of the drugs recommended in this book.

British Library Cataloguing in Publication Data
A catalogue record for this book is available from the British Library

Library of Congress Cataloging-in-Publication Data
A catalog record for this book is available from the Library of Congress

ISBN-10   0 340 815 736
ISBN-13   978 0 340 815 731

1 2 3 4 5 6 7 8 9 10

Commissioning Editor: Clare Christian
Project Editor: Clare Patterson
Production Controller: Jane Lawrence
Cover Designer: Nichola Smith

Typeset in 9/11 Minion by Charon Tec Pvt. Ltd, Chennai, India
www. charontec.com
Printed and bound in Malta

What do you think about this book? Or any other Hodder Arnold title?
Please send your comments to www.hoddereducation.com

In memory of Gurlal and Manjit Massi

Contents

Preface

'Employ your time in improving yourself by other men's writings, so that you shall gain easily what others have labored hard for.'

Socrates (469–400 BC)

Writing a second edition is a first for me, and therefore to maintain proximity to the subject matter I recruited the help of my younger brother, whom I thank dearly. This second edition comes after five years and contains many necessary additions, deletions and refinements. However, the text remains succinct and true to its original objectives with an emphasis on aiding memory.

During this period the MRCPsych examination has altered considerably and will no doubt evolve further. It is therefore essential that prospective candidates obtain the most recent College guidelines and familiarize themselves with the syllabus. Knowing what you are up against is part of the equation, but equally important is timely preparation.

Chuff, chuff, chuffing the train comes,
Everybody gets up and quickly runs,
Pushing and shoving and squeezing through,
Just in time before the whistle blew.

Gin aged 9

Boarding a train is very much like passing an examination. Only some people will be able to make the journey and in order to do so you need to know your destination, possess a valid ticket, and have the good sense to be on the correct platform in time. The key to success lies in thorough planning and preparation that requires due diligence to detail. The basic sciences outlined in this book are essential knowledge for appreciating the biological and psychological underpinnings of psychiatry, and learning can be greatly enhanced by taking an interest in the subject matter.

A cursory glance through this book would suggest that we have made major advances since the time of Socrates; however, many would argue that we have barely moved. Either way, I hope that by using this book you will 'gain easily what others have labored hard for' and that the knowledge you gain will be of benefit beyond your immediate goal.

Gin S. Malhi

Acknowledgements

We thank the doctors at all levels of psychiatry training who have provided feedback over the last few years. We also thank our own teachers and mentors and in particular those that we learn from most, our patients.

Basic psychology

LEARNING THEORY

Learning is the acquisition of knowledge or skill that is not the result of maturation. It can take place through association, understanding or observation.

1 Associative learning includes classical and operant conditioning.
2 Cognitive learning involves understanding and uses cognitive strategies to process information.
3 Observational learning involves modelling.

ASSOCIATIVE LEARNING

CLASSICAL CONDITIONING (CC) (RESPONDENT LEARNING)

Described by Pavlov (1849–1936) in 1927, who trained dogs to salivate in response to a light or bell by associating it with food.

CC involves repeated administration of a new stimulus (bell) together with an **unconditioned stimulus** (UCS) (food).

The UCS (food) is known to elicit a specific **unconditioned response** (UCR) (salivation).

This repeated association results in the new stimulus (bell) being able to produce the same response (salivation), eventually without the UCS (food).

The new stimulus (bell) is the **conditioned stimulus** (CS) and the learned response it produces (salivation) is now termed the **conditioned response** (CR), once the association has been acquired.

The forming of an association is an **automatic behaviour** (passive process) and does not require understanding. It can be regarded as a means of extending a response from one stimulus to another. So, for example, in Pavlov's experiments the dogs' response of salivating to food was extended to a bell.

The period of pairing required between an UCS and a CS for the association to be learned and the conditioned response to occur is called the **acquisition stage**.

Acquisition of a CR is selective and the fact that certain stimuli are more likely to become a CS than others is termed **stimulus preparedness**.

In **simultaneous conditioning**, the CS and UCS are applied together (CS continues until response occurs). This is less effective than **delayed conditioning**, in which the start of the CS precedes the start of UCS (optimal delay is less than 1 s). Least effective is **trace conditioning**, in which the CS ends before the UCS begins.

If the CS is repeatedly presented without the UCS then the CR gradually disappears, though usually not completely. This is called **extinction**.

If there is then a period during which the CS is not presented, the CR may return in a weakened form. This is termed **partial** or **spontaneous recovery**. The CR can also be recovered by repeating the association with the UCS.

Learning to respond to a new CS through association with the original CS (but not the original UCS) is **higher-** or **second-order conditioning**. If a stimulus similar to the CS is used, the response is **generalized** and enables learning of similarities. Response generalization diminishes in proportion to the degree of dissimilarity between the new stimulus and the original CS.

Discrimination is the ability to recognize and respond to the differences between similar stimuli and can be produced by differential reinforcement.

For emotional reactions, repeated brief exposure to the CS can result in a large increase in the strength of the CR. This is termed **incubation**.

In 1920, **Watson and Rayner** used CC to induce a white-rat phobia in **Little Albert** (11-month-old boy) by associating a loud noise with every presentation of the rat. This was then repeated with a white rabbit, and eventually the boy's fear was generalized to any furry object.

OPERANT CONDITIONING (OC) (INSTRUMENTAL LEARNING)

Skinner (1904–1990) proposed an associative learning theory based on **Thorndike's** (1874–1949) **law of effect**. This states that if a voluntary behaviour (operating on trial and error) is rewarded it will be repeated, and vice versa.

A hungry rat placed in a Skinner box (contains a lever which releases food pellets) learns to press the lever in order to receive food. In this way the CR (pressing the lever) is reinforced. Operant conditioning is thus an active form of learning (the rat must act in order for conditioning to occur).

Primary reinforcement rewards basic drives (e.g. nourishment, sex) and is independent of prior learning.

Secondary reinforcement rewards learned drives (e.g. money, praise) and is more subjective.

Reinforcement can be **positive**, whereby a reward reinforces a response and increases the likelihood of its occurrence, or **negative**, whereby an unpleasant condition is removed and again increases the likelihood of the response (e.g. patient-controlled analgesia). **Punishment** is an aversive consequence that is intended to reduce the likelihood of recurrence, and is most effective when given promptly. The removal of a punitive measure may allow it to act as a negative reinforcer.

Punishment is one of three kinds of **aversive conditioning**. The other two are **avoidance conditioning**, in which the conditioned response prevents an adverse event occurring (seen in obsessive–compulsive disorders), and **escape conditioning**, in which the CR provides escape from the adverse event (seen in phobias; extremely resistant to extinction). When performed in the imagination aversive conditioning is termed **covert sensitization**.

In operant conditioning, different **schedules of reinforcement** lead to varying behavioural patterns. This is known as programming.

With **continuous reinforcement** (contingency reinforcement) every positive response is rewarded. The behaviour is quickly acquired and the response rate is at its maximum.

In **partial reinforcement** only a fraction of the responses are reinforced. Behaviours learned by this method can be very resistant to extinction (variable > fixed). Types of schedule are:

- *fixed interval* reinforcement (reward follows a fixed amount of time) is relatively poor at maintaining a CR and the response rate only increases at expected time of reward
- *fixed ratio* reinforcement (reward follows fixed number of responses) is effective in maintaining rapid response rate
- *variable interval* reinforcement (reward follows a continually varying amount of time regardless of the number of responses) is effective in maintaining a CR
- *variable ratio* reinforcement (reward follows a continually varying number of responses) produces a relatively constant rate of response.

A common example of operant conditioning techniques is the **token economy** (Allyon and Azrin). This is often used in behavioural management programmes for children, in which a desired behaviour is rewarded with stickers or tokens which can then be swapped for privileges.

In **chaining**, a desired behaviour is broken down into a series of simpler steps which are then taught separately and eventually linked together.

Shaping is also based on operant conditioning, and involves reinforcing successively closer approximations to a desired behaviour so that it is eventually achieved satisfactorily. Like chaining, it can be useful for people with learning difficulties.

Premack's principle states that a high frequency behaviour can be used to reinforce a lower frequency one by making engagement in the former contingent upon satisfying some aspect of the latter.

In **reciprocal inhibition** (Wolpe, 1958) the connection between an anxiety-inducing stimulus and its response (i.e. anxiety) is weakened by the concurrent administration of an anxiety-inhibiting stimulus. The theory is that opposing emotions cannot exist simultaneously (though some researchers dispute this).

This then forms the basis of **systematic desensitization**, used in the treatment of phobias, which involves graded exposure (in imagination or reality) to the anxiety-inducing stimulus along a previously decided **hierarchy** (from mild to severe). Immediate exposure to stimuli at the top of the hierarchy without any prior gradation is called **flooding** when carried out *in vivo* and **implosion therapy** when imagined.

Habituation is a form of adaptation that involves learning not to respond to frequent stimuli of little consequence.

Sensitization is another form of adaptation where the strength of a response is increased because of the (perceived) significance of the stimulus (i.e. the opposite of habituation).

COGNITIVE LEARNING

This is an active form of learning that involves the creation of cognitive maps and the development of structure and meaning.

Cognitive learning takes place either as **insight learning** (spontaneous cognitive remodelling that provides a sudden insight or solution to a problem) or **latent learning** (learning occurs but is not immediately apparent).

OBSERVATIONAL LEARNING [VICARIOUS/IMITATION/SOCIAL LEARNING (ASSOCIATED WITH BANDURA), MODELLING]

This is an active form of learning that takes place through observation. It may lead to the occurrence of both classical and operant conditioning, but there is no direct reinforcement.

Relevant characteristics of those being observed:

- share features with observer (similarity)
- have a high status
- perceived competence
- their behaviour is seen to be rewarded.

Another factor is the observer's perceived self-efficacy; their confidence in their own ability to perform.

PERCEPTION

This is the conscious awareness and interpretation of sensory information. It is an active process that improves with learning and maturation, and is intrinsically linked with the attribution of meaning.

The Weber-Fechner law relates the strength of a stimulus to how intensely it is perceived. Visual and auditory perception have been studied the most.

GESTALT PRINCIPLES OF PERCEPTION

- Visual phenomena:
  - **continuity:** interrupted line perceived as continuous (e.g. table edge partially obscured behind a chair)
  - **closure:** incomplete outline perceived as whole (e.g. biscuits on a plate are perceived as intact despite overlapping and obscuring each other)
  - **proximity:** juxtaposed items grouped together (e.g. || || || is perceived as three pairs of lines rather than six individual lines)
  - **similarity:** grouping of items that look alike
  - **simplicity:** preference given to most basic percept possible based on the available information.
- Perception of the whole differs from that of its individual components ('the whole is greater than the sum of its parts').

FIGURE GROUND DIFFERENTIATION

Ability to distinguish a stimulus (e.g. an object or sound).

OBJECT CONSTANCY

Ability to perceive an object as being the same despite varying viewing conditions.
  Several kinds:

- colour/lightness constancy: object colour and lightness remain constant irrespective of lighting
- size constancy: object size perceived as constant irrespective of distance
- shape constancy: object shape perceived as constant irrespective of perspective (angle)
- location constancy: object position perceived as constant irrespective of viewer's motion.

PERCEPTUAL SET

The tendency to perceive on the basis of expectation. It includes:

- a reduction in threshold for expected percepts, and vice versa
- distortion/modification of ambiguous percepts in order to fit with expectation.

Influencing factors: personality, experience, emotion.

DEPTH PERCEPTION

To create 3D perception from 2D retinal images the brain relies on several cues:

- monocular accommodation
- binocular vision and convergence
- object interposition
- object texture gradient
- linear and aerial perspectives
- relative size and brightness
- elevation and motion parallax.

DEVELOPMENT OF VISION

Development of visual perception is dependent on interaction with the environment (constitutional–environmental interaction):

- *birth*:
    - can discriminate levels of brightness
    - able to fix objects
    - able to track and scan objects

– figure–ground discrimination
– fixed focus (0.2 m)
- *1 month*: differentiate faces; preference shown for complex stimuli
- *2 months*: possess depth perception
- *4 months*: colour vision and accommodation
- *6 months*: accurate acuity (6:6).

(NB: Perceptual constancy, depth perception and object completion are acquired abilities and not present at birth.)

INFORMATION PROCESSING

This spans everything between sensory input and perception. Early stages include perceptual set, object constancy and figure–ground differentiation. Processing is mostly unconscious and progresses in stages of organization and interpretation. It can be data driven or conceptually driven.

DATA-DRIVEN PROCESSING

Prompted by data arrival. Utilizes pre-established templates for pattern recognition and classification.

CONCEPTUALLY DRIVEN PROCESSING

Insufficient data are extrapolated into a probable percept. Evidence is then sought in support of this possibility.

ATTENTION

The selection of information for further processing. There are several kinds:

FOCUSED (SELECTIVE) ATTENTION

A single stream of information is selected for attention. **Dichotic listening** experiments show that alternative information is simultaneously processed and can be attended to if required.

DIVIDED ATTENTION

Simultaneous attention is given to more than one source of information. Inefficient performance because of **dual-task interference**.

CONTROLLED ATTENTION

Requires effort.

AUTOMATIC ATTENTION

Practice makes tasks increasingly automatic.

SUSTAINED ATTENTION

Performance progressively deteriorates.

STROOP EFFECT

Interference of conscious process by deeply rooted automatic processing (e.g. saying the actual colour of the following word: WHITE). Stroop effects are used in frontal lobe assessment (a disinhibited individual has difficulty suppressing an automatic response).

MEMORY

Specific memories may be highly localized, but the processes of memory are not.
   Memory is intrinsically linked to learning and involves:

- acquisition of skills and associations
- storage of information
- learning of new information (anterograde memory)
- recall of previously learnt information (retrograde memory).

MEMORY PROCESS

- Registration of information
- Storage of information
- Retrieval of information.

REGISTRATION/ENCODING

The initial processing of information that enables it to be analysed (requires attention).

STORAGE

1 **Multi-store or dual-memory model** (Atkinson and Shiffrin). Sensory, short- and long-term systems.
      Sensory memory Large capacity but information is unanalysed, unconscious and of very short duration. Sense-specific: *echoic* – auditory (up to 2 s), *iconic* – visual

(0.5 s) and *haptic* – touch. Sensory memory bridges the finite resolution of the senses, allowing discrete data to be 'joined' together for further processing (e.g. we perceive rapidly changing still images as moving television pictures).

Short-term memory (STM) (primary/working memory) Temporary memory that allows conscious processing of information. Fades rapidly (within 20 to 30 s) unless rehearsed, typically by repetition. Coding is primarily acoustic. Purely visual STM is very brief, and visual information is typically translated into acoustic code (e.g. repeating written lists or telephone numbers out loud).

Finite capacity (7 ± 2 units of information) that can be increased by **chunking** (Miller, 1956), which is the expansion of one unit to incorporate several more by introducing a meaning, link or formula between them. Visual and verbal STM are stored in the R and L hemispheres respectively. Recall is error-free and effortless.

Long-term memory (LTM) (secondary memory) Permanent store. Theoretically unlimited capacity. Requires a few uninterrupted minutes for consolidation. Regardless of presentation, information is stored and organized systematically and subsequent loss through forgetting is slow. Coding is primarily (but not exclusively) semantic and requires motivation. Storage and retrieval require effort.

LTM is either **declarative** (expressed through language and sub-divided into episodic and semantic) or **procedural** (expressed through action). Declarative memories are experienced explicitly (recalled completely with subjective temporal awareness). Procedural memory is *IMP*licit (no conscious recollection or temporal awareness) and concerns skills (*I*ntuition, *M*otor, *P*erception).

Episodic An **autobiographical memory** for events and places.

Semantic (knowledge) Vocabulary, meanings, significance.

2   An alternative is the **levels of processing model** (Craik and Lockhart). From superficial to deep, the levels are: sensory, phonetic, semantic. STM and LTM are regarded to be processes rather than the structures of the Atkinson and Shiffrin model. The deeper the level of processing, the stronger the trace-strength (i.e. the deeper the 'impression' the stimulus leaves) and the more likely the information will be retained.

RETRIEVAL

The recall of information from memory (LTM $\rightarrow$ STM).

Emotion influences retrieval:

* facilitated by positive emotion because of increased rehearsal and organization
* impaired with negative emotions/anxiety
* facilitated by reproducing original emotional context (**state-dependent learning**).

Primacy and recency effects Accurate recollection of an item is more likely if it is one of the first or last items to be learnt. Primacy occurs because initial items receive most consolidation and recency because immediate information is still in STM.

Forgetting is more often a failure to access information than to retain it.

HYPOTHESES OF FORGETTING

Interference theory New learning disrupts the recall of a previously learned item because it interferes with the consolidation of that item (**retroactive inhibition**).

Conversely, prior learning can interfere with subsequent learning (**proactive inhibition**). Forgetting is item dependent.

Decay theory Memories fade with time (trace-strength diminishes). Information in STM is lost before being transferred to LTM, or information from LTM is lost if it is not used for a long time.

Repression Deliberate (motivated) forgetting.

Displacement If the STM is 'full', new information displaces old information.

MOTIVATION

Motivational theories attempt to explain behaviour in terms of cause (needs) and effect (the resulting acts). There are several dimensional approaches to classification (conscious vs. unconscious, innate vs. learned, internal vs. external).

Needs produce drives which in turn motivate behaviour intended to meet those needs (goal-seeking behaviour). Needs – physiological, can be defined objectively. Drives – psychological, acquired.

Primary (physiological/homeostatic/innate) drives Necessary for survival. Arise from biological need. For example, ablating the hypothalamic ventromedial nucleus (HVN) causes hyperphagia (hence HVN designated as the satiety centre), while ablation of lateral hypothalamus (hunger and thirst centre) causes aphagia.

Secondary (acquired/non-homeostatic) drives Develop in association with secondary needs (subjectively determined goals) through stimulus generalization and conditioning (i.e. they are learned). Vary considerably between individuals (e.g. anxiety is a secondary drive).

Two main theories of drive, both requiring extrinsic (environmental) input:

1 **Cannon's homeostatic drive theory** Change in homeostatic system triggers processes aimed at restoring equilibrium (i.e. they self-regulate). Basic (biological) needs function homeostatically. To meet these intrinsic needs requires extrinsic elements (e.g. thirst requires water).
2 **Hull's drive-reduction theory** Hull argued that all behaviour was ultimately driven by primary needs and based on learning (i.e. interaction with the environment). Mowrer and others later expanded Hull's ideas to include secondary drives.

In intrinsic theories of motivation, internally motivated behaviour is regarded to be sufficiently gratifying or rewarding in itself without necessarily requiring external interaction, though this may still occur.

1 **Festinger's cognitive dissonance theory** Incompatible cognitions, or beliefs inconsistent with behaviour, cause dissonance which the individual is motivated to resolve by altering one of the parameters (cognition, belief or behaviour). The desire for cognitive consistency can therefore be considered a need (see Chapter 2).
2 **Need for achievement (McLelland)** Need for achievement (cognitive model of motivation) relates to 'need' for self-ideal. Failure to match ideal results in drive to achieve. Eventual mastery results in pleasure, is intrinsically rewarding and involves

desire for stimulation (as opposed to homeostatic mechanisms which are designed to reduce stimulation). Can be achieved through personal **COMPE**tence:

Curiosity
Others (cooperation, reciprocation)
Manipulation
Play
Exploration.

3 **Arousal theory** Individuals are usually motivated to achieve the optimal level of arousal at which they will perform best. Excessively high or low levels of arousal lead to sub-optimal performance, though with familiar (well-practised) tasks a high level of arousal is generally optimal, and vice versa (**Yerkes–Dodson curves**).

Maslow's (1908–1970) hierarchy of needs combines extrinsic and intrinsic elements.
Ordered according to survival value. Those that are lower in the hierarchy must be at least partially satisfied before subsequent (higher) needs can be addressed:

7 **Self-actualization**
intrinsic motivations, altruism
6 **Aesthetic**
symmetry, beauty, order
5 **Cognitive**
understanding, exploration, knowledge
4 **Esteem**
social approval, competence, recognition
3 **Belonging and love**
affiliations, relationships
2 **Safety**
protection, security
1 **Biological**
air, food, water, shelter

EMOTION

A feeling is the experience (i.e. awareness) of a bodily sensation (touch, heat, pain, movement etc.) or an emotion. An emotional state can be regarded as a combination of the prevailing physiology, thoughts and behaviour. It defines the context of subjective experience. Several theories of classification, but generally all agree on a certain core of emotions (universal) from which all others can be derived (culturally diverse). Amygdala has a central role in biology of emotion.

Robert Plutchik's classification is based on eight primary emotions, which he represented on the inside of a wheel. The degree of emotion is variable (represented by the arrows), and combining any two adjacent primary emotions gives rise to a secondary emotion (e.g. surprise + sadness = disappointment). Love/remorse and disappointment/optimism are regarded to be mutually exclusive polar opposites, as shown in the following diagram:

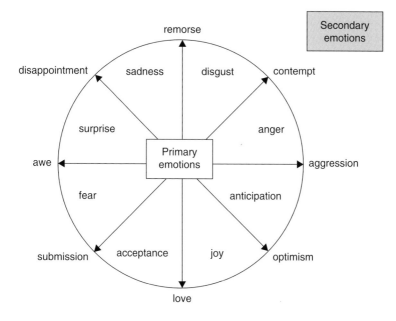

JAM*ES*–LANGE THEORY (1922)

Perception of an emotion-arousing stimulus causes physiological changes which are then mentally interpreted and experienced as the relevant emotion. The emotion is therefore secondary to physiological response.

Criticisms:

* emotional changes faster than physiological response
* pharmacological induction of physiological states not accompanied by appropriate emotion
* same physiological response can occur with different emotions
* emotions can be independent of physiological response.

SCHACTER'S COGNITIVE LABELLING THEORY

Schacter also believed emotions were secondary to physical arousal, but that their nature was determined by cognitive appraisal. In other words, physiology merely generates the 'energy' of emotion, which must then be directed (or labelled) by thought. Studies have shown that similar circumstances and physiological reactions can be variously emotive according to the cognitive appraisal of the situation.

CANNON–BARD (THALAMIC) THEORY

Perception of an emotion-arousing stimulus leads to the concurrent experience of emotion and physiological response. Thalamus controls processing of sensory information and stimulates both the cortex (to produce the appropriate feeling) and the viscera (via hypothalamus, to produce the relevant physical reaction). An important feature of this theory is that the feeling and biological aspects of emotion are processed independently but at the same time.

STRESS

Strictly, any activity (physical or mental) which requires significantly more effort than baseline (to either execute or endure) is 'stressful'. In human psychology, the term is usually restricted to situations where demands (stressors) exceed resources. These two variables are subjective, which is why individuals' stress may differ despite (objectively) similar circumstances.

Like any emotion, stress comprises feelings, physical changes and cognitions which are a reaction to the situation.

SITUATIONAL FACTORS

Examples are life events, daily hassles or uplifts, conflict, emotional and physical trauma. Life events (LEs) are those which disrupt one's routine or way of being (can be positive or negative). They are therefore stressful (subjectively determined) and so can be attenuated by such factors as social support. Negative LEs have been shown to be positively associated with illness (as predisposing, precipitating or maintaining factors) across all cultures.

PHYSICAL ASPECTS

Non-specific (i.e. anything stressful elicits the same physical response). Described by Hans Selye as the General Adaption Syndrome:

- initial alarm (fight or flight)
- resistance (state of increased arousal)
- exhaustion (with chronic stress).

Stress can cause or exacerbate many illnesses (e.g. heart disease, peptic ulceration). Physical illness may itself be a stressor.

PSYCHOLOGICAL ASPECTS

Negative stress is either directly or indirectly associated with almost every class of psychiatric disorder, particularly the mood and neurotic disorders. Conversely, positive LEs can alleviate morbidity.

1 **Reaction to stressors determines susceptibility to illness**
  Type A personalities (relatively more vulnerable): *DISTRAC*tible

  *D*riven
  *I*mpatient
  *S*trive for *S*uccess
  *T*ime urgency
  *R*arely *R*elax
  *A*mbitious
  *C*ompetitive

  NB relationship between type A personality and coronary heart disease.
  Type B individuals perceive changes/stressful events as challenges and have a greater sense of control over their lives.

2 **Coping mechanisms**
  Conscious responses employed to counter stress. Problem-focused responses attempt to modify stressor. Emotion-focused responses attempt to modify individual's reaction.

3 **Locus of control**
  Rotter identified two dimensions of perceived control over life:

  Internal locus Feeling of being in control of one's life and responsible for personal behaviour. This is associated with a healthy response to stress.
  External locus The opposite, i.e. feeling that life is externally controlled and 'out of one's hands'. This is associated with a poor response to stress.

4 **Learned helplessness**
  Learned generalized helplessness, the belief that nothing will work or make any difference; illustrated by Seligman using dogs. Forms part of cognitive model of depression.

Social psychology

ATTITUDES

Acquired ways of relating to particular individuals, groups or ideas. They:

1 define social groups
2 establish identities
3 influence thought and behaviour.

Attitudes have several specific functions: **SKIVE**:

Social adjustment – facilitate sense of belonging to a community
Knowledge – facilitate understanding of the world
Instrumental – practical or pragmatic
Value-expressive – express values
Ego-defensive – preserve self-esteem and shield from anxiety.

Attitudes predispose an individual to behave in a particular manner. They comprise three components (**A,B,C**):

an **A**ffective component – feelings towards attitude object
a **B**ehavioural component – actual response/interaction with attitude object
a **C**ognitive component – beliefs concerning attitude object.

In theory, these components influence each other and are mutually consistent. However, because of situational variables (e.g. wanting to 'look good' or avoid 'looking bad') they may not predict behaviour. Attitudes tend to predict behaviour best when they are:

1 strong and consistent
2 based on subject's personal experience
3 related specifically to the predicted behaviour.

MEASUREMENT OF ATTITUDES

Direct methods of measurement:

1 **Thurstone scale**: uses statements that have been ranked and assigned values by a panel. Subject selects those they agree with. Disadvantages: bias in ranking; different responses can result in same overall score.
2 **Likert scale**: subject indicates degree of agreement/disagreement on a five-point scale for each of a number of different statements. More sensitive than Thurstone scale but different responses can still result in same overall score.
3 **Semantic differential scale**: paired opposites (e.g. 'strongly agree' and 'strongly disagree') are placed at either end of a line along which subjects are free to mark their response, which can then be measured as the distance along the line. Easy to use and has good test–retest reliability. However, difficult to interpret midpoint responses and there may be positional response bias.

Direct measures are susceptible to social desirability bias: subject offers expected answers as opposed to genuine responses. Lie scales can detect the likelihood of this happening, and the tendency can be diminished by emphasizing anonymity or embedding questions within apparently irrelevant items.

Indirect methods can be used to assess attitudes but interpretation is difficult: physiological responses (e.g. Galvanic skin response); projective tests (e.g. Rorschach inkblot, thematic apperception and sentence completion tests).

Other important methods for assessing attitude:

* *Borgadus social distance scale*: measure of racial prejudice. It involves selecting statements from a range that represents varying degrees of social distance
* *Sociometry*: subjects in a group nominate preferred partners for a particular task/friendship, the results of which can be represented as a sociogram (a network of preferred relationships) that helps identify sub-groups
* *Interview*: open-ended or structured.

ATTITUDE CHANGE

Generally very difficult. May focus on the behavioural (e.g. reward/punishment) or cognitive aspects of attitude. Affective component most resistant to change.

Cognitive consistency theories link attitudes so that the way we respond to one affects the way we respond to another. May also be regarded as theories of motivation.

1 **Heider's balance theory**: individuals seek harmony of attitudes and beliefs and evaluate related things in similar manner.
2 **Festinger's cognitive dissonance theory**: when an individual's actions are inconsistent with their attitudes this produces dissonance, prompting a change in attitudes so they fall in line with behaviour. Dissonance is a negative drive state, characterized by psychological tension/discomfort, producing increased arousal that the individual attempts to reduce by:
    – altering behaviour
    – dismissing dissonance creating information (i.e. ignoring/denying it)

  – developing and adding new explanations or ideas in favour of thoughts that are
    consonant.
  Attitude change is also a means of reducing dissonance.
    The degree of dissonance is in proportion to the perceived importance of the
    cognitions involved.
    Increased dissonance occurs when:
  • there is little pressure to comply
  • the perceived choice is high
  • there is an awareness of personal responsibility for any consequences
  • consequences of any alternative behaviour are anticipated to be unpleasant.
  Predictions of this theory are counter-intuitive, imprecise and only partly
    supported empirically.
3 **Osgood and Tannenbaum's congruity theory**: when two attitudes or beliefs are
  mutually inconsistent, the one that is less firmly held will change.

PERSUASIVE COMMUNICATION

Persuasion is dependent upon characteristics of the source (communicator), the message
and the audience (recipient). Applies to many situations, e.g. doctor–patient interactions, advertising etc.

PERSUASIVE COMMUNICATORS

Possess a *RANGE* of characteristics:

• *R*ecognized opinion leader
• *A*udience is able to identify with communicator through similarity and/or com-
  municator is *A*ttractive/likeable
• *N*on-verbal cues facilitating communication (e.g. optimal proximity to audience)
• *G*enuine motivation and having no vested interest in message
• *E*xpertise and credibility.

RECIPIENT FACTORS (i.e. audience characteristics)

• *Intelligence*: curvilinear relationship.
• *Self-esteem*: when low the use of simple messages enhances compliance. Complex
  messages are persuasive in intelligent recipients with high self-esteem.

MESSAGE

*I*mplicit message more persuasive for *I*ntelligent recipient, explicit message more
effective for less intelligent recipient.

Interactive personal discussion more persuasive than impersonal one-way mass media communication.

One-sided uncritical presentation better suited to less intelligent audience and those who already favour message.

Two-sided presentation better suited to well-informed and intelligent audience, particularly if neutral towards message.

Fearful message better at influencing recipients with low levels of anxiety, and the converse applies to those with high levels of anxiety (low fear message is better).

Type of persuasion determines kind of **attitude change**:

- *Identification* based on attraction to/admiration of communicator.
- *Internalization* based on belief in the message.
- *Compliance* based on punishment/reward and not really a change of attitude.

INTERPERSONAL ATTRACTION

Individuals seek others for support, friendship and companionship. Interpersonal attraction, a facet of interpersonal perception, is enhanced by several factors: *PARCELS*:

Proximity/Propinquity: dependent upon degree of intimacy and culture-bound interpersonal space
Attractiveness (physical)
Reciprocal self-disclosure
Competence (perceived)
Exposure (familiarity), i.e. how long individuals spend together
Liking (reciprocal)
Similarity: particularly significant in early stages of a relationship.

Complementarity does become more important as relationship progresses, but does not supersede similarity.

THEORIES OF INTERPERSONAL ATTRACTION

Exchange theory: preference for relationships that offer greatest gains (reward) with least expense (cost).

Equity theory: additional factors of investment and constancy are considered in gauging rewards and costs of a relationship. The relationship should be 'fair' with approximately equal gains in the long run.

Proxemics: interpersonal space (body buffer zone) is determined by personal factors and cultural rules and mediated by non-verbal cues. Different body parts vary in terms of availability for contact (gender and relationship of those involved is also important): hands > arms/face > trunk/legs > pelvic region.

Some individuals have larger personal space, e.g. schizophrenics and violent criminals (particularly behind themselves). Initially respond violently to intrusion of this and then withdraw.

Matching hypothesis (similarity hypothesis): pairing of individuals (to form romantic partners) results in them being closely matched in terms of their mutual rewards. Usually, a partner of similar physical attractiveness is sought.

ATTRIBUTION THEORY

Attribution is the process of interpreting the behaviour of others/oneself. It is a cognitive process concerned with determining behavioural causality on the basis of observed behaviour.

Types of information that can be used to make attributions: (Kelley)

Consensus, Consistency and Distinctiveness

Individuals tend to attribute their own behaviour to situational (external) causes but that of others to dispositional (internal) causes. This bias in attributing the behaviour of others is called the **fundamental (primary) attribution error**.

SELF

An individual's **self** or **self-concept**, as described by Carl Rogers, consists of all the perceptions, values, attitudes and ideas they have concerning themselves. It does not necessarily reflect or correspond to reality. Separate from this is the **ideal self**, which is all that the individual would like to be.

SOCIAL INFLUENCE

SOCIAL FACILITATION

Task performance is enhanced by the presence of others. Facilitation is not necessarily because of competition; others can simply be observers (**audience effect**, Dashiell).

However, with new or complicated tasks, or hostility from others, performance may decline.

Bibb Latane proposed a *S*ocial *I*mpact *T*heory (*SIT*) stating that in any particular setting the degree of social influence is a function of the:

*S*trength,
*I*mmediacy and
*T*otal number of people exerting the influence.

In social situations of urgency **bystander intervention** is impeded by **pluralistic ignorance** (looking to others for a reaction) and **diffusion of responsibility** (denial of personal responsibility).

SOCIAL POWER

Influence over others exerted by individuals or a group. Five methods/types are described by French and Raven: *RACER*:

   Reward: influence is derived from being able to reward
   Authority: (legitimate) influence is derived from status or role
   Coercion: influence is derived from ability to punish (usually implied)
   Expertise: influence is gained by demonstrating skills or knowledge
   Referential: influence is because of charisma, being liked and admired.

CONFORMITY

Yielding to group pressure by way of persuasion or example such that there is a change in attitude or behaviour.

   Informational social influence: individual conforms to group ideas and behaviour outwardly and privately.

   Normative social influence: conforms outwardly but privately maintains own opinion.

   Solomon **Asch**: used confederates (accomplices, stooges) in small groups to attempt to alter the opinion of an individual assessing which line was longer relative to another. Naïve subject shown to be significantly influenced by confederates' incorrect answers.

   To avoid social rejection the subject agrees with the group view even when their own personal opinion differs.

   Conformity increases with:

- group number (maximum effect with **three** confederates)
- perceived high status of other group members.

NB conformity diminishes greatly if even a single member of the group agrees with subject.

   Vulnerability to conform is less in those that are:

- self-reliant
- intelligent
- socially able
- expressive.

OBEDIENCE

Milgram (Stanley) conducted experiments involving the apparent administration of electric shocks by subjects, under the instruction and supervision of an 'expert' (experimenter), to protesting individuals who were in fact part of the experiment and acting accordingly (i.e. stooges). He was able to show that the subject's obedience was **increased** by:

- perceived authority of experimenter
- presence of experimenter

- belief in 'contract' with experimenter
- distancing from distressed and protesting individual.

Subject's obedience stems from:

- acceptance of experimenter's sense of right and wrong
- inability to challenge experimenter's morality because of ensuing social awkwardness.

Zimbardo (Philip), using college students in a mock prison, similarly showed that unwillingness to express moral concerns could lead to tolerance of escalating brutality.

LEADERSHIP

Leadership characteristics dependent upon:

- task requirements
- group characteristics
- development (pathway to becoming a leader)
- influence ascribed by role.

Distinction of three **LeAD**ership styles and their effect on groups (Table 2.1) (Lewin, Lippitt and White, 1939):

> **L**aissez-faire
> **A**utocratic
> **D**emocratic

Table 2.1 Leadership styles

	Laissez-faire	Autocratic	Democratic
Interaction within group	Aggressive	Aggressive	Cooperative, friendly, show initiative, responsibility
Interaction with leader	Detached	Submissive, dependent, attention-seeking	Task-related
Absence of leader	Abandon task	Abandon task	Continue independently
Task completion	Poor	Good	Good
Most effective for	Creative tasks	Urgent tasks	Routine tasks

Fiedler's contingency theory: Fiedler (Fred) correlated leadership style (measured using LPC, see below) with task and group characteristics.

Degree to which leaders distinguish between least and most preferred co-workers gives rise to a 'least preferred co-worker' (LPC) scale.

High LPC score: leader is **relationship orientated** and perceives least preferred co-worker quite favourably. Considerate and accepting in relationships.

Low LPC score: leader is **task orientated** and strongly disapproves of least preferred co-worker. Dominant and controlling in relationships.

The theory proposes that high and low LPC leaders are suited to different types of tasks, and that this is influenced by their relationship with the group (see Table 2.2).

Table 2.2 Contingency theory

Task	Relationship with group	Best leader
Structured	Good	Low 'least preferred co-worker'
Unstructured	Good	High 'least preferred co-worker'
Unstructured	Poor	Low 'least preferred co-worker'

GROUPS

Group decisions tend towards consensus, with individuals suppressing opposing opinions so as to avoid dissension. This is described as **groupthink**, and results in inadequate exploration of alternatives. It occurs in situations where there is:

- pressure to complete a task
- a prominent opinionated leader
- a cohesive group shielded from outside influence.

If individuals express their opinions separately first, and then as a group decide upon the same matter, the eventual outcome is likely to be more extreme than that of the group average. This is termed **polarization** and occurs partly because of reinforcement.

Within groups the individual behaviour of the members is less important than that of the whole group. This suppression of individuality is termed **deindividuation**.

Ingroup: any group with which a person identifies.

Outgroup: any group with which the person has an association but does not identify.

Group membership: leads to biases of social perception:

- outgroup is perceived as being homogenous*
- ingroup is perceived as being heterogeneous*
- members of ingroup are perceived more positively (Tajfel's **social identity theory**).

(*NB reciprocal applies if ingroup is the minority group).

Prejudice: a biased attitude (i.e. one that cannot be wholly supported by objective evidence). Discrimination, the application of prejudice, can occur on the basis of any attribute, e.g. sex (sexism), race (racism), age (ageism).

Explanations for prejudice:

- *Cultural*: competition between groups for common resources results in cohesion within the groups and inter-group hostility (realistic conflict theory)
- *Motivational*: frustration from one source is displaced and expressed as aggression (authoritarian personality; frustration-aggression theory)
- *Cognitive*: development of defective beliefs about other groups (stereotyping).

To reduce prejudice there should be (Cook):

- an environment supporting equality
- the attainment of equality
- the opportunity for inter-group contact
- contact with non-stereotypes
- collaborative endeavour.

Stereotyping: assigning a particular group's perceived characteristics (real + imagined) to individuals regarded to be from that group. Stereotypes form the cognitive component of prejudice. Once established, they are difficult to change and become self-fulfilling, in that fresh observations are biased by the working stereotype and only supportive information is selected.

AGGRESSION

Behaviour intended to intimidate.
   Instrumental aggression: aim is to cause a desired outcome.
   Hostile aggression: aim is to inflict suffering.

THEORIES OF AGGRESSION

Ethological theories: Aggression is innate. Behaviour that diminishes aggression:

- distancing self from aggressor
- familiarity with aggressor
- evoking conciliatory response.

   Operant conditioning: the consequences of aggression determine the likelihood of repetition. Gains (physical, psychological, social) act as positive reinforcers.
   Psychoanalytical theories: consider aggression to be a basic instinct.
   Social learning theory: aggression is learned through modelling (i.e. observation).
   Frustration–aggression hypothesis: failure to achieve causes frustration. Frustration is intimately linked with aggression, and aggressive drive precipitates aggressive behaviour. Emotional arousal increases aggressive behaviour, possibly through classical conditioning. Aggression can be directed towards the source of frustration or displaced. Although frustration usually leads to aggression, it can instead cause emotional disturbance or apathy.
   Media: viewing television violence increases aggressive behaviour in boys (social reinforcement).
   Correlates of aggressive behaviour: characteristics of parents and family associated with an individual's aggressive behaviour:

- Family: large
            lower socio-economic group
            lack of positive emotional expression

- Parents: young; aggressive
            physical punitive measures
            inconsistent or permissive in parenting.

INTERPERSONAL COOPERATION

Altruism: helping behaviour in which the interests of others are given importance above one's own. Strictly applied there should not be any perceived personal gain. Generally, helping behaviour is not completely unselfish. Altruism is regarded by some as a defence.

Social exchange theory: behaviour is driven by the expectation of reward. Regarding helping behaviour, the expectation is that of future reciprocity.

Interpersonal cooperation: Cooperation usually applies in circumstances where:

- without cooperation a specific aim cannot be fulfilled
- another party also has the same aim
- the aim is not exclusive (i.e. can be fulfilled simultaneously by more than one party).

In such situations cooperative behaviour is influenced by:

- number of parties involved (with increasing numbers cooperation diminishes)
- prior knowledge of other parties
- behaviour of other parties
- extent of communication between parties
- perceived pros and cons of various actions undertaken.

Neuropsychology

This is the study of mental processes from a biological perspective.

DYSPHASIA

Dysphasias are an impairment of language processing. They may be expressed in writing and/or gesture, but are usually described in terms of their manifestation in speech (the aspects of which are outlined in Table 3.1).

Although the prefix *a-* usually means 'absence of' and *dys-* 'impairment of', this rule is not always followed. For example, individual dysphasias (e.g. Broca's) are commonly referred to as aphasias.

Terms such as **anomia** (inability to name objects; seen in most dysphasias), **agrammatism** (loss of grammar), **acalculia** (acquired difficulty with certain arithmetical operations), **dyslexia** (impaired reading), **agraphia** (inability to write) etc. describe particular difficulties and are not usually specific diagnoses, though they may occur in isolation.

The presence (and severity)/absence of these signs is used to help build up a picture of a subject's particular dysphasia. Similarly, fluency is a non-specific sign of dysfunction posterior to the sylvian fissure (or lateral sulcus), e.g. Wernicke's aphasia (converse is true for non-fluent speech, e.g. Broca's aphasia).

Around 95 per cent of R-handed and 70 per cent of L-handed individuals show left hemisphere dominance for language. The area around the left sylvian fissure is broadly regarded to be the language area of the brain, though many other areas are additionally involved with language processing.

Table 3.1 Dysphasias

Term	Explanation	Location in L hemisphere
Semantics	Meaning of words	Temporal lobe
Phonology	Language sound-pattern	Superior temporal
Syntax	Grammar	Anteriorly
Prosody	Intonation; emotional content	Anteriorly right* hemisphere

* exception.

The peri-sylvian area includes aspects of the frontal, parietal and temporal lobes. The location and extent of damage determine type of dysphasia, and clinically there is often overlap. The right hemisphere governs prosody (intonation of speech; the insertion and interpretation of emotional inflexions).

PERI-SYLVIAN DYSPHASIAS: REPETITION IMPAIRED

- *Broca/motor/expressive*: lesion in the inferior frontal gyrus (opercular/triangular zones, BA 44 and 45, anterior language zone), which coordinates the expression of speech. Subject experiences a discrepancy between what they are going to say and what they actually say. Speech reveals a level of understanding but is broken (NB 'Broca'), hesitant and effortful, as if attempting to communicate in a second language.

  Agrammatism → telegraphic speech. Words may be substituted by sound or meaning (phonemic and semantic paraphasias respectively). Deficits are usually partial. Comprehension remains intact, though ability to write is often affected. Subject is frustrated by their inability to communicate. [After Broca, Paul (1824–1880).]
- *Wernicke/sensory/receptive*: lesion in the superior temporal gyrus (auditory association cortex, BA 22 and 42, posterior language zone), which makes sense of language. Subject is unable to correctly translate their thoughts into language and vice versa, impairing both their comprehension and communication skills.

  Speech is fluent but incoherent, and may include neologisms (if frequent this is sometimes called jargon aphasia). Naming is profoundly impaired. Writing and reading are also affected. Subject has limited awareness of their language deficit. [After Carl Wernicke (1848–1905).]
- *Conductive*: damage to supramarginal gyrus close to arcuate fasciculus, the main connection between Broca's and Wernicke's areas. Sometimes occurs during recovery from Wernicke's aphasia. Subjects occasionally try to correct their paraphrasic errors. Comprehension and verbal fluency unaffected, but repetition severely impaired.

TRANSCORTICAL (EXTRA-SYLVIAN) DYSPHASIAS: REPETITION INTACT

Most commonly associated with the *watershed infarction*; involves the borderline cortical areas supplied between the terminal tributaries of the major arteries. A more anterior infarction implicates Broca's area = transcortical motor dysphasia; a more posterior lesion implicates Wernicke's area = transcortical sensory dysphasia. These can be further subdivided.

Transcortical dysphasias are not just a peri-sylvian dysphasia with repetition relatively intact (though this is a helpful simplification); they have other differentiating features.

SUBCORTICAL DYSPHASIAS

There is debate as to whether isolated lesions in subcortical areas produce distinct dysphasias. The issue is not whether these areas are involved with language (they clearly are) but whether they actually perform part of the processing, or instead connect and coordinate the other (cortical) processing centres.

Recovery tends to be better with these dyphasias. This may be because subcortical areas perform a largely supportive role in language that can be partially compensated if compromised, rather than a highly specialized role that cannot.

- *Thalamic*: dominant thalamus lesion, esp. pulvinar nucleus. Features include anomia and $\downarrow$ verbal fluency with relatively good comprehension and repetition.
- *Basal ganglia*: hemiparesis is accompanied by difficulties with comprehension and dysarthria.

GLOBAL APHASIA

Seen in infarctions of the left middle cerebral artery, affecting most of the language area. Subject is unlikely to be able understand or express any language. Partial recovery is possible, usually towards a Broca's-type dysphasia as there may be a right cortical redundancy for understanding language, but not for its expression (which is more localized to the left).

NEURONAL CIRCUITS

1   Speech → auditory association → Wernicke's area → comprehension.
2   Mentation → Wernicke's area → Broca's area → motor regions → speech.
3   Text → visual association → angular gyrus → Wernicke's area → comprehension.
4   Mentation → Wernicke's area → angular gyrus → motor regions → writing.

OTHER CORTICAL COGNITIVE FUNCTIONS

Agnosias and apraxias often occur together, particularly with left-hemisphere lesions.

AGNOSIA

An inability to recognize something; to interpret sensory information despite intact sensory pathways. Agnosias occur with lesions in cortical association areas.

- *Visual*: inability to interpret visual information. Contrast with anomia, in which subject is unable to name objects but knows what they are and can describe their use. Visual agnosics can do neither.

  Sub-divided into apperceptive (subject finds it difficult to perceive, i.e. to integrate basic optical information such as form, perspective, angles etc. into a coherent visual experience) and associative (subject can perceive visual information but does not understand it, i.e. objects have no meaning).

  These subdivisions can also be applied to other sensory modalities (e.g. auditory associative agnosia). Types of visual agnosia include: simultagnosia (subject is able to grasp the individual aspects but not the overall meaning of a picture); prosopagnosia (inability to recognize familiar faces).

- *Autotopagnosia*: a form of 'body-specific representation disorder', in which the subject has difficulty identifying their own body parts. Invariably occurs with somatotopagnosia (difficulty in identifying another's body parts), though this latter term is not commonly used.
- *Agraphagnosia*: inability to identify numbers/letters traced on the skin. Also called agraphaesthesia/graphanaesthesia.
- *Phonagnosia*: impaired recognition of familiar voices.
- *Finger agnosia*: inability to identify individual fingers; seen in Gerstmann's syndrome.
- *Astereognosia*: inability to recognize objects by touch. Sometimes called tactile agnosia.
- *Hemisomatognosia*: a form of unilateral spatial neglect (usually seen following a right hemisphere stroke).
- *Anosognosia*: failure to recognize, or denial of, hemiplegia.
- *Topographic agnosia*: inability to orientate oneself in a familiar environment. A characteristic feature of Alzheimer's disease, it is an aspect of non-dominant parietal lobe dysfunction.

APRAXIA

Loss of an ability to perform a motor task (*as if* the subject has forgotten how), despite intact motor and sensory systems.

- *Verbal apraxia/motor aphasia*: an inability to coordinate the articulation of certain words, particularly difficult or unfamiliar words, despite intact motor function. Contrast with dysarthria, which is the poor articulation of all speech due to impaired motor function.
- *Constructional*: a somewhat 'catch-all' term (i.e. not just apraxias) for disorders that result in an inability to draw/copy/construct shapes or structures.
- *Ideational*: inability to coordinate a sequence of movements to perform a task.
- *Oral/buccofacial*: inability to perform certain movements with the lips/tongue, e.g. whistle, wag tongue from side to side etc.
- *Ideomotor*: inability to mime an action or activity, e.g. sawing a piece of wood.

FRONTAL LOBES

Frontal cortex of humans is uniquely enlarged and the most recently developed part. The frontal lobes make up a third of cerebral hemispheric mass. Specific areas:

- *motor area*: pre-central gyrus (sensory area = post-central gyrus = parietal lobe)
- *pre-motor area*: anterior to motor area (BA 6 and 8)
- *dorsolateral area* (BA 9, 10, 45, 46)
- *basomedial area* (BA 9–13, 24, 32).

Dorsolateral and basomedial areas are often grouped together as prefrontal region/cortex. Frontal eye field is a specialized area located in posterior portion of middle frontal gyrus (BA 8).

DISORDERS INVOLVING FRONTAL LOBES

- Neoplasms: 90 per cent of brain tumour patients presenting with psychiatric symptoms have frontal lobe involvement
- Cerebrovascular diseases
- Multiple sclerosis
- Trauma
- Degenerative diseases.

MOTOR AND PRE-MOTOR CORTEX

- Function
  - motor control (primary and secondary levels)
  - fluency (verbal and design)
- Lesion effects
  - motor: contralateral spastic paresis; loss of fine motor control
  - fluency: reduced (particularly verbal)
  - spelling: impaired
- Others: *GROUPS*:
  - *G*egenhalten (opposition)
  - *R*eflexes (primitive)
  - *O*ptic atrophy (ipsilateral)
  - *U*rinary incontinence (bilateral damage)
  - *P*erseveration (failure of response inhibition)
  - *S*eizures (Jacksonian).

PREFRONTAL CORTEX

- Intellectual functions: *SPACE*:
  - *S*equencing (ordering tasks)
  - *P*rocessing (mental agility)
  - *A*ttention
  - *C*oncentration
  - *E*xecution.

Any of these can be impaired in frontal lobe damage.

- Personality changes:

pseudopsychopathic *CDEFGH*	pseudodepressive *RAPID*
[orbitofrontal damage]	*[dorsolateral damage]*
*C*hildish excitement (**moria**)	*R*etardation (psychomotor)
*D*isinhibition	*A*pathy
*E*uphoria	*P*lacidity
*F*amiliarity	*I*ndifference (lack of concern)
*G*arrulousness	*D*iminished *D*rive (lack initiative)
*H*umorous punning (associated with moria).	

FRONTAL LOBE TESTS

Frontal lobe tests have increasingly come to be known as executive tests, in recognition of the fact that executive functionality is not restricted to the frontal lobes. The associated impairments are called dysexecutive signs/symptoms.

Executive functions are those that allow a person to reflect on and adapt their interaction with others and with the environment. A dysexecutive syndrome (formerly frontal lobe syndrome) is not a fixed entity; it may comprise a variety of different executive impairments, the range and severity of which will vary from one individual to another.

The following is not an exhaustive list of frontal tests, nor are the tests necessarily specific for frontal impairments.

ABSTRACTION

- *Proverb interpretation*: ask subject to explain up to three well-known proverbs, e.g. 'People in glass houses shouldn't throw stones'. Initially they can be encouraged to give a free interpretation, which can be assessed for its degree of 'concreteness'. If this fails, the subject can be given four possible interpretations and asked to choose the correct one.
- *Similarities*: e.g. What's similar about an apple and a banana?/table and chair? The pairings become progressively more abstract, e.g. television and magazines?/music and painting? Healthy subjects approach the question from a categorical perspective (e.g. fruit, furniture, entertainment, art), whereas those with frontal impairment give very literal similarities (e.g. you can eat them, they have four legs, you look at them, they are fun).
- *Cognitive estimates*: subjects are asked to guess the answers to 10 to 15 questions (in a clinical exam a few will usually suffice) that do not depend on knowledge or deduction, e.g. 'How many camels are there in France?' or 'How long is the average man's leg?' Answers are scored as normal, slightly extreme, extreme or very extreme (in comparison with controls).

INITIATION

Verbal fluency: subject must list as many words as they can beginning with F, A and S (one minute for each letter), avoiding proper nouns, repetitions or words with the same root (e.g. run, runs, running etc.). Young professionals' total combined score <30 abnormal, elderly with poor education <25 abnormal. Healthy subjects should not perseverate or revert to a previous letter.

Subjects can also be asked to list as many animals as possible (an example of a semantic category) in 1 minute (beginning with any letter): 20 is usually normal, 12–15 is in lower acceptable range (depending on age/education).

RESPONSE-INHIBITION AND SET-SHIFTING

- *Alternating sequences*: examiner asks the subject to copy a pattern of alternating squares and triangles beyond the original drawing:

The impaired subject will tend to perseverate, repeating either the square or the triangle design rather than alternating them.

- *Motor sequencing*: the Luria 3-step test involves demonstrating a sequence of hand movements – fist, edge, palm – five times (without any verbal commentary) and asking the subject to repeat the sequence.

    In the alternating hand movements test, the examiner opens and closes his hands alternately (i.e. left hand open + right hand closed, then vice versa, and so on). The subject is then asked to copy this movement.

- *Wisconsin card-sorting test*: subject is asked to sort a pack of cards with different symbols/colours/patterns into particular categories which must be worked out by feedback from the tester. For example, when the subject places a red square alongside a red circle the examiner says no, but when he places a black circle next to the red circle the examiner says yes; hence the category in this case is shape, not colour, and the subject would be expected to proceed accordingly. The categories are continually changed during the course of the test.

- *Trail-making test*: 'joining the dots', e.g. 1, 2, 3 … 10 or 1, a, 2, b, 3, c … and so on. There are various versions of this test.

- *Glabellar tap*: tapping on the forehead of a healthy subject will result in a degree of habituation of the blink reflex (i.e. blinking is eventually inhibited). This is impaired in those with frontal deficits.

MOTOR CONTROL

- *Primitive reflexes*: palmo-mental, grasp, pouting, sucking.
- *Utilization behaviour*: subject repeatedly uses objects within their grasp but does so inappropriately or out of context, without insight into their behaviour; e.g. picking up somebody else's cup, stapling a piece of paper etc.
- *Imitation behaviour*: subject mimics the actions of others without insight into their behaviour.

Psychological assessment

4

PRINCIPLES

A good test should be:

- reliable
- valid
- discriminatory
- standardized.

It should preferably be:

- easy to administer
- cost-effective.

SCALING

This involves the classification of information in accordance with a scale. The scale is based on some characteristic of the information.

Structurally different scales:

- *Nominal*: qualitative information; categories of classification; not suited to statistical analysis. Individual units of information have no relative value or hierarchy. Group can be described by mode, frequency or proportion
- *Ordinal*: scores are ranked and have relative but not absolute value, signifying order but not the degree of difference. Group can be described by range and median
- *Interval*: ordinal scale with scores separated equally. No absolute zero but uniform intervals allow derivation of both order and difference. Group can be described by arithmetic mean and variance
- *Ratio*: akin to interval scale with uniform intervals but in addition possesses an absolute zero; values therefore have an absolute value (i.e. not just relative to each other). Group can be described by geometric mean and coefficient of variation.

Scales can also be classified according to purpose:

- *Discriminatory (differential)*: provide groups or categories. Can be used for classification or diagnosis
- *Descriptive (intensity)*: measure extent or severity
- *Prognostic*: measure course and outcome
- *Selection*: predict outcome following specific treatment.

METHODS OF ASSESSMENT

RATINGS SCALES

- *Respondent* (self-report): e.g. Zung Depression and Anxiety scale, Beck Depression Inventory (BDI), Michigan Alcohol Screen Test, Hospital Anxiety and Depression Scale, Minnesota Multiphasic Personality Inventory (MMPI), Holmes and Rahe Social Readjustment Rating Scale (for life events), General Health Questionnaire.
- *Interviewer* (or observation): e.g. Hamilton Depression Rating Scale (HAM-D; not valid in physically ill as several items likely to be confounded), Positive and Negative Symptom Scale (PANSS), Brief Psychiatric Rating Scale (BPRS), Health of the Nation Outcome Scale (HONOS), Clinical Global Impression, Global Assessment Scale, Montgomery and Asberg Depression Rating Scale.

ERRORS OF ASSESSMENT

- *Central tendency*: bias towards centre, avoiding extremes.
- *Leniency error*: tendency to select extremes.
- *Response set*: consistent tendency to either agree or disagree with questions.
- *Logical error*: rating items that have some 'logical link' in a similar fashion (treating them as a group).
- *Hawthorne effect*: presence of interviewer alters the situation and influences responses, i.e. knowledge of the observation influences the observation.
- *Halo effect*: answers are selected so as to fit with other responses.
- *Social acceptability*: respondent gives expected answers (those believed to be expected/wanted by interviewer). Can be reduced by use of forced-choice or false items.

NORM-REFERENCE

A standard score for a group/population is termed the norm. New results are then compared with this norm. This approach allows the results from different studies to be compared both to the population norm and to each other.

CRITERION-REFERENCE

This serves a similar purpose to norm-referencing. However, the standard (i.e. the criterion) is selected more arbitrarily, often chosen such that comparison allows assessment of performance on a particular test. Criteria should be unbiased, reliable and relevant.

VALIDITY

The extent to which a test/scale measures what it is supposed (or claimed) to measure.

- *Content validity*: degree to which all aspects of the relevant subject are assessed.
- *Face validity*: whether the intended characteristic appears to be measured (subjective appraisal).
- *Criterion validity*: ability of test or measure to distinguish between subjects already known to differ on the basis of an external, validated test. Two types:
  - *concurrent validity*: comparison of test result(s) with those of another prevalidated measure
  - *predictive validity*: ability of test to predict the outcome as determined later by another (established) scale.
- *Cross validity*: extent to which the validity of a measure is retained when applied to a new set of subjects.
- *Incremental validity*: extent to which a new measure improves on previous measures (i.e. how much 'better' it is).
- *Construct validity*: relates to the purpose of the measure and relies on establishing:
  - *convergent validity*: degree of association between measures that are expected to be closely correlated (correlation is assumed because they measure the same property)
  - *divergent validity*: degree to which a measure discriminates between that which is being assessed from unrelated measures.

RELIABILITY

The reliability of a test/measure indicates the degree to which it can be 'trusted', i.e. to what extent the results can be replicated. The more reliable a test, the more consistent its result(s) (given the same test conditions).

- *Inter-rater reliability*: degree of agreement between different raters assessing the same parameters within the same time-frame.
- *Intra-rater reliability*: degree of agreement between assessments made at different times by the same raters assessing the same parameters.
- *Split-half reliability*: assesses the internal consistency of a test/measure; the extent to which equivalent components (two halves) of the test/measure correlate when compared.
- *Test–retest reliability*: assesses the stability of a test/measure; the degree of correlation between two assessments conducted under identical conditions but at different times.

INTELLIGENCE

Various definitions based on different parameters can be used to define and describe intelligence. No single definition is universally accepted, and no single test for overall 'global intelligence' (though many psychologists agree global intelligence is a valid concept).

- *Galton*: attempted to measure intellect.
- *Spearman*: developed concept of **g**eneral intelligence factor (**g**).
- *Thurstone*: proposed primary mental abilities: **MNOPQRS: M**emory, **N**umber, w**O**rd fluency, **P**erceptual speed, verbal **Q**omprehension, **R**easoning, **S**pace.
- *Hebb*: type A (genetically-based potential), type B (effective intelligence).
- *Cattell*: fluid ability (used for novel situations/problems; basis of initiative and creativity) and crystallized ability (relies on prior learning and use of previous experience/knowledge).
- *Sternberg*: component intelligence (deductive ability and verbal reasoning; used for executive tasks) and experiential intelligence (automation of routine tasks, permitting attention to be focused on new learning).

Intelligence is best categorized according to what is being assessed: **ABCD**

Assessment

- *psychometric methods*: define and examine specific and general abilities, e.g. visual and verbal factors of intelligence. Performance correlates between specific factors, but it is difficult to say how many factors there should be (i.e. how many aspects there are to intelligence).
- *computational methods*: examine the information processing involved in problem solving. Five components suggested (Sternberg): **TRAMP: T**ransfer; **R**etention and **A**cquisition components, which deal with transfer of knowledge, memory and learning; **M**eta-components, which decide upon selection of strategies; and **P**erformance components, which carry these out.

Biological aspects e.g. heritability, diet
Cultural aspects e.g. emphasis on education/learning
Developmental aspects e.g. degree of stimulation in formative years.

Attainment: achievement; consequence of learning.
Aptitude: potential ability.
Intelligence quotient (IQ): percentage ratio determined by mental age (MA; measure of intellectual ability devised by Binet) and chronological age (CA): IQ = (MA/CA) × 100.

Assessments designed such that average MA score equals CA, providing a mean IQ of 100 (standard deviation 15). Intelligence assumed to have a normal distribution (see Chapter 18).

Measured intelligence increases up to 16 years of age, then plateaus from 16 to 25 years, followed by gradual decline until 5 years prior to death, when there is a *terminal drop*.

INTELLIGENCE TESTS

ADULTS

Wechsler Adult Intelligence Scale (WAIS) [revised (WAIS-R)]: for those aged 16 years and over. Consists of 6 verbal and 5 performance subtests, providing verbal and performance IQs.

Verbal: SAD VIC

Similarities
Arithmetic
Digit span
Vocabulary
Information
Comprehension

PerfOrmance: *ABCD*

Object assembly
picture Arrangement
Block design
picture Completion
Digit symbol

Scores are summed to provide overall IQ. Performance scale more sensitive to normal ageing than verbal scale. A large difference between verbal and performance scores renders overall test interpretation invalid.

Halstead-Reitan Neuropsychological Battery (HRNB): for ages 15 and over. Designed to be a comprehensive neuropsychological assessment, typically in cases of brain damage. Comprises 10 individual tests and the possible addition of WAIS and/or MMPI.

National Adult Reading Test (NART): estimates pre-morbid IQ using lists of words with difficult/obscure pronunciation. Not a direct measure, but pronunciation has been shown to be positively correlated with intelligence.

Mill Hill Vocabulary Test: based on recognition and recall.

Raven's Progressive Matrices: involves diagram completion. Different tests for different age groups. Does not rely on recall and easy to use; less sensitive to cultural differences and can be used for those with communication difficulties. Measures aptitude.

CHILDREN

Stanford–Binet Intelligence Scale: from 2 to 15 years. Tests short-term memory and reasoning (verbal, quantitative, abstract, visual). IQ is derived by comparison with normative data.

Wechsler Pre-school and Primary School Intelligence Scale (WPPSI): from 4 to 6½ years. Verbal and non-verbal.

Wechsler Intelligence Scale for Children (WISC) [revised (WISC-R)]: from 5 to 15 years. Verbal and non-verbal.

Reitan-Indiana Neuropsychological Battery for children: from 5 to 8 years.

Halstead Neuropsychological Battery for children: from 9 to 14 years.

INTELLIGENCE TESTS AFFECTED BY:

- individual factors: anxiety, motivation
- situational factors: interaction with assessor (e.g. hostility)
- test factors: age specificity (children especially), function/purpose specificity.

CONTENTIOUS FINDINGS CONCERNING INTELLIGENCE

- Inappropriate use has led to erroneous interpretations, e.g. IQ variance according to racial differences.
- Intelligence has an inverse relationship with:
  - increasing family size
  - birth order.
- Positive associations:
  - inheritance (of intelligence)*
  - education.
  (*Heritability of intelligence is a controversial issue; however, the closer the biological relationship the closer the IQs approximate.)
- Studies show that IQ of children is related to:
  - home lifestyle
  - education
  - perseverance.

NB not particularly related to parental wishes or social class.
Boys have greater range of intelligence than girls.

PERSONALITY ASSESSMENT

Nomothetic (nomological) theories: based on population studies and concerned with the structure of personality (trait and type theories).

Ideographic (radiological) theories: based on study of the individual and concerned with aspects of individuality (personal construct, humanistic and psychoanalytic theories).

Bannister's repertory grid: uses bipolar constructs to assess attitudes.

CATEGORICAL VERSUS DIMENSIONAL APPROACHES TO PERSONALITY

Categorical approach places people in distinct categories (e.g. Kretschmer's and Sheldon's associations with body-build). Dimensional approach characterizes personality in terms of extent/intensity of traits (e.g. Eysenck's and Cattel's theories, which are examples of nomothetic theories).

Kretschmer: Linked personality and body-build as follows:

- *athletic* (muscular): outgoing, robust
- *asthenic/leptosomatic* (lean): solitary, self-conscious, cold, aloof, self-sufficient, schizothymic
- *pyknic* (rounded and stocky): relaxed, sociable, cyclothymic, variable in mood.

Sheldon made similar types of links:

- *mesomorphy* (muscle, bone): somatotonia, show energy and assertiveness
- *ectomorphy* (fragility): cerebrotonia, prefer symbolic expression
- *endomorphy* (soft, roundness): viscerotonia, prefer enjoyment, relaxation.

Eysenck's personality theory: derived four dimensions from factor analysis of rating scale data: neuroticism–stability; extroversion–introversion; psychoticism–stability; intelligence.

Cattel's trait theory: derived three dimensions from 16 personality factors (PF) which in turn were derived from an analysis of thousands of words describing personality (first 12 PF based on ratings of one person by another; last 4 based on data from self-ratings): intelligence, anxiety, sociability (similar to Eysenck's dimensions).

Measurement: Maudsley Personality Inventory (MPI); Eysenck Personality Inventory (EPI) and Eysenck Personality Questionnaire (EPQ). Latter is a recent development; it assesses psychoticism and contains a lie-scale.

PSYCHOMETRIC ASSESSMENT OF PERSONALITY

Objective: e.g. EPQ, MMPI. Respondent has limited options. Mental state significantly interferes with scoring; hence semi-structured interviews and observer-based ratings preferred.

Projective: based on presenting an ambiguous stimulus to which the individual then responds, e.g. Thematic Apperception, Rorschach Inkblot, sentence completion and draw-a-person tests.

Human development

5

STAGE THEORIES

Development occurs as a series of progressive stages. Each is necessary for the occurrence of subsequent maturation. The sequence of stages is constant and environmental influences can only alter the rate of development. Transitions between stages are described as **critical periods**.

Progression through stages and critical periods is driven by **maturational tasks**. These tasks allow the development of more complex behaviours. The culmination of developmental processes is termed **maturity**, which can be described more specifically as physical, intellectual or sexual maturity.

ATTACHMENT

John **Bowlby** coined the term 'attachment' to describe a child's connection to its mother (*bonding* is mother's connection to child; *engrossment* is father's connection to child). The seeking of social contact (*sociability*) is seen as a basic dimension of temperament and a pre-requisite for attachment.

Attachment behaviour is that displayed by the infant towards the **attachment figure** (the focus of such behaviour), from whom affection, comfort and warmth are sought even in preference to food (**Harlow**'s monkey experiments).

Bowlby described four phases to normal (healthy) attachment:

- *Pre-attachment* (0–2 months): preference for human rather than environmental comfort
- *Attachment in the making* (2–8 months): infant increasingly responds to primary caregiver only. When one individual is chosen (usually the mother), this is termed **monotropic** attachment (usually seen at 6 months)
- *Clear-cut attachment* (8–24 months): uses caregiver as base and protests at their departure. Emergence of fear of strangers at 12 months
- *Goal-directed partnership* (from 2–3 years): begins to understand caregiver's goals/ motives. Learns trust (caregiver is reliable), reciprocity (relationships are two-way)

and effectance (what they do affects the relationship). Attachment figure can be temporarily substituted, provided needs of child are adequately met.

Bowlby regarded an infant's attachment with its mother to be primary. This view has been criticized, notably by the work of Schaffer and Emerson (1964), who showed that a large proportion of children do not display monotropy and do not have primary attachments with their mother but with other family members (e.g. father).

Lorenz explained attachment as a form of **imprinting**, which occurs in animals other than primates (the animal forms an attachment to the first adult it sees).

SECURE ATTACHMENT BEHAVIOUR

Prominent during first three years of life (6–36 months). Lays foundation for initiative and formation of relationships.

- Attachment figure (AF) separation causes distress and anxiety.
- Upon return of AF infant seeks contact/comfort from AF.
- Infant uses AF as secure base from which to explore environment, returning intermittently to seek reassurance and comfort.

Secure attachment depends upon:

- temperament of infant
- AF nurturing
- AF encouraging independent exploration
- AF providing secure base.

Separation before 6 months or after 3 years of age has little effect. This then is the critical period during which separation leads to:

- protest: crying and searching for AF
- despair: as AF has not returned
- detachment: indifference to AF.

Prolonged separation (maternal deprivation) is associated with: ***ABCDE***

- *A*ttention-seeking and *A*ggressive behaviour
- *B*onds are difficult to make and sustain (easily *B*roken)
- *C*old, un*C*oncerned behaviour
- *D*evelopmental language delay and *D*warfed growth
- *E*nuresis.

INSECURE ATTACHMENT BEHAVIOUR

	Avoidant	**Ambivalent**
In absence of AF	muted clinginess	excessive anxiety
Upon return of AF	little or no reaction	unsure of whether to engage

Insecure attachments may lead to disorders of childhood and adolescence and difficulties in establishing relationships. Avoidant attachment may lead to aggressive behaviour later in life.

Mary **Ainsworth** (1913–1999) conducted two important studies on attachment, the first in 1967 in Uganda and the second in 1971 in Baltimore, USA. Both involved interview (of the mother) and observation (of the child). The Baltimore study made use of a standard measure of attachment behaviour she had helped devise called the **Strange Situation**, in which eight scenarios were enacted in a room in the following sequence with a 1-year-old baby:

> Mother + baby introduced into room → mother + baby in room
> (3 min) → stranger + mother + baby (3 min) → stranger + baby
> (≤3 min) → mother + baby (≥3 min) → baby
> (≤3 min) → stranger + baby (≤3 mins) → mother + baby (3 min).

The adults in each scenario have a specific role to play (e.g. be silent, interact with each other, interact with the baby). The flexibility of timing is to allow for variations in infant behaviour. Greater emphasis is placed on infant's reaction to mother's return than to her departure, as this is thought to be a clearer indicator of attachment.

Ainsworth classified the infants into three groups: Group A, **anxious-avoidant** (20 per cent); Group B, **secure** (70 per cent); Group C, **anxious-ambivalent** (10 per cent), and demonstrated a strong positive correlation between these groups and **maternal sensitivity** to the infant (i.e. her ability to correctly interpret and respond to the infant's signals).

Mary **Main** has studied attachment over the longer term, both in children and adults. In 1991 she and others devised and used the **Adult Attachment Interview**, a semi-structured psychoanalytic-type interview (what is said given less emphasis than how it is said) of early attachment history. She too defined three groups, which mirror those of Ainsworth: Group D (**detached**), Group E (**enmeshed**), Group F (**autonomous**).

FAMILY RELATIONSHIPS

PARENTING

Involves various components described as:

- nurturance (P → C)
- communication (P ↔ C)
- control (P → C)
- maturity demands (P → C).

Parenting style can be categorized as:

- authoritative: nurturing parents with high expectations and strict rules
- authoritarian-restrictive: less nurturing but still controlling
- permissive: unconditionally nurturing.

Different styles of parenting result in different characteristics of children.

DISTORTED FAMILY FUNCTION (DYSFUNCTIONAL FAMILIES)

Exhibit: *CORE*

Communication problems
Overprotection: of members of family, aspect of enmeshment; excessively close
Rejection: weak attachments within family and parents under-involved; loneliness
Enmeshment: over-involved parents stifle child's individuality.

Exclusive relationships within the family (triangulation) can also cause discord, as can scapegoating children for marital discord.

INTRAFAMILIAL ABUSE

Most damaging in early childhood as this is time of greatest vulnerability and developing personality. Abuse can be physical, sexual or both.
Sequelae common to both forms of abuse:

- depression and anxiety states
- dissociation
- disordered personality (particularly borderline personality disorder)
- distrusting and paranoid traits
- dependence on defence mechanisms (denial, splitting).

PHYSICAL ABUSE (NAI – NON-ACCIDENTAL INJURY)

Sequelae:

- are themselves aggressive, may suffer impairments (neurological, cognitive) and delays in development
- are likely to repeat abusive behaviour towards own children.

SEXUAL ABUSE

Sequelae: *SHAME*

Sexual impulses more difficult to control and sexual identity is weakened
Homosexuality is more likely
Alcohol and drug abuse
Molestation of children is more likely
Eating disorders (this is disputed).

Abuse (physical and sexual) in the long term causes diminished self-esteem and a predisposition to self-harm.

DIVORCE

Parental divorce is almost invariably associated with some degree of distress to children. Usually this is self-limiting (up to a year) and outcome is dependent on:

- child's temperament and age at time of divorce
- nature of the divorce (amicable, hostile)

- relationships between siblings and between children and parents
- degree of communication
- parents' abilities to adjust and make provisions for the children.

TEMPERAMENT

Temperament refers to the basic dimensions of personality (sociability, emotionality, activity) thought to have a biological basis and appear early in life.

The New York Longitudinal Study (Thomas and Chess, 1977–1984) studied the interactions of children and their parents, and grouped them as follows:

- *Easy child (40 per cent)*
  - regular in habits (eating, sleeping)
  - adaptable to change/novel situations
  - emotional stability
  - positive and responsive to new stimuli.
- *Difficult child (10 per cent)*
  - irregular in habits
  - slow or unable to adapt
  - emotional lability
  - negative and unresponsive to novel stimuli.
- *Slow-to-warm-up (40 per cent)*
  - slow to adapt
  - suspicious of novel situations
  - poor response to new stimuli, often withdrawn.

A fourth group could not be easily categorized.

THEORIES OF DEVELOPMENT

PIAGET (COGNITIVE MODEL)

Jean Piaget (1896–1980), having observed his own children, proposed that a child's cognitive development is dependent upon interaction with the environment and progresses at varying rates through specific stages. Children think differently (qualitatively) to adults and are often unable to distinguish or separate their personal perspective (**egocentrism**). Intelligence involves understanding and inventing new ways of interacting with the environment.

Schema: cognitive structure or pattern of behaviour/knowledge.
Assimilation: incorporation of new or novel information into existing thought patterns (i.e. schemas).
Accommodation: adjustment or modification of existing schemas to facilitate comprehension of new information.

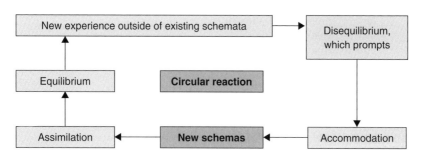

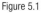
Figure 5.1

Therefore, as shown in Figure 5.1:
   Piaget described four stages (NB ages are approximate):

1   **Sensorimotor stage (0–2 years)**: child has innate reflexes that are modified by
   functional exercise. Develops causal relationships between self and outside world.
   Does not understand temporal relationships and exhibits egocentrism
   – *4 months*: primary decentring; detaches self from external environment. Develops
     discriminatory smiling
   – *8 months*: purposeful behaviour commences
   – *12 months*: begins to develop object permanence (i.e. hidden object still exists).
2   **Pre-operational stage (2–7 years)**: pre-causal logic; animism; symbolic stage.
   – Child uses deferred imitation (symbolic play, drawing) and acquires compo-
     nents of language. Thought involves: *AMPLE* ('ample thought')
   – *A*nimism: characteristics of life are attributed to all objects
   – authoritarian *M*orality: rules are sacrosanct, bad-doing should inevitably be
     punished
   – *P*recausal *L*ogic: non-scientific, based on child's internal world
   – *E*gocentrism
   – Occasionally divided into **pre-conceptual** (2–4 years) and **intuitive** (4–7 years).
3   **Concrete operational stage (7–11 years)**: myelination of the CNS is complete at age
   7 years. Children lose animism, authoritarianism and egocentrism. A second decentring of thoughts occurs, enabling development of logical thought. Able to perform
   operations such as those involved in comprehending the **laws of conservation**.
   Aspects of thought that take prominence are: *LOGIC*

      *L*ogic
      *O*perations (mental manipulation of thoughts)
      *G*roup activity/cooperation
      *I*dentity and *I*ndividuation of thought (but understand other person's point
      of view)
      *C*omprehend *C*onservation (reversibility).

4   **Formal operational stage (11 years and upwards)**: beginning of hypotheticode-
   ductive thought, involving the complex manipulation of ideas and the application
   of sophisticated reasoning: *ABCD*

*A*bstract (propositional) thought
*B*elief systems
*C*onceptualization
*D*eductive reasoning.

NB this stage may not necessarily be attained even by adulthood.

KOHLBERG (MORAL DEVELOPMENT)

Kohlberg proposed six stages of moral development, grouped in three levels, derived from posing moral dilemmas to a variety of subjects.

Level I: pre-conventional morality
- stage 1: punishment
- stage 2: reward

Level II: conventional morality
- stage 3: approval/disapproval
- stage 4: authority

Level III: post-conventional morality
- stage 5: social contract
- stage 6: personal principles/ethics

Though there is some correlation between age and morality, many adults may not reach level III. Levels I and II can be loosely correlated to Piaget's preoperational (2–7 years) and concrete operational (7–11 years) stages respectively. Level III is usually begun in adolescence.

Social perspective-taking is the ability to adopt 'another person's point of view'; i.e. be objective and detach opinion. It is a precursor of empathy and moral reasoning. Prerequisites are adequate cognitive and moral development and a robust sense of personal identity.

MARGARET MAHLER (DEVELOPMENT OF SENSE OF SELF)

Used psychoanalytic theory; focused on how self-identity is established.

- *Normal autistic phase* (0–4 weeks): establishes an equilibrium with environment.
- *Normal symbiotic phase* (4 weeks–5 months): exists as part of caregiver (symbiote).

The sub-phases of separation-individuation:

- *First (differentiation) sub-phase* (5–10 months): begins to differentiate between self and non-self (i.e. caregiver, environment); stranger anxiety
- *Second (practising) sub-phase* (10–16 months): begins to explore non-self, practising separation; separation anxiety
- *Third (rapprochement) sub-phase* (16–24 months): reacting against non-self, wanting to fuse (re-approach) with mother; ambivalence/frustration

- *Fourth (object constancy) sub-phase* (24–36 months): ↑ independence; mother can be trusted to be there if needed.

FREUD (PSYCHOSEXUAL DEVELOPMENT)

See Chapter 7.

ERIK ERIKSON (PSYCHOSOCIAL DEVELOPMENT)

Extends into adulthood. Requires the successful resolution of a crisis at each phase of development (see Table 5.1). Erikson emphasized concepts of identity (inner sense of self); identity crisis and identity confusion. Epigenesis refers to the stages of ego and social development.

Table 5.1 Psychosocial development (NB Ages double) (cf. Freud's psychosexual stages of development)

Age	Crisis	Successful outcome
0–18 months	Trust/mistrust	Sense of security/attachment
18–36 months	Autonomy/doubt	Self-control/efficacy
3–6 years	Initiative/guilt	Confidence
6–12 years	Competence/inferiority	Competence
12–adulthood (adolescence)	Identity/confusion	Achieve self-identity
Adulthood	Intimacy/isolation	Commitment
Middle-age	Generativity/stagnation	Concern about others
Maturity	Integrity/despair	Fulfilment

Erikson (1902–1994) adopted Freud's structural and topographical models and agreed that development is biological, i.e. genetically determined, but disagreed with psychosexual emphasis. Freud emphasized Id; Erikson emphasized Ego.

KELLY'S PERSONAL CONSTRUCT THEORY

Man's interpretation of the world is scientific. Based on personal experience, each individual formulates various constructs that allow them to make predictions. Each individual's system of constructs, both conscious and unconscious, is organized in a hierarchy and provides a sense of identity. Having to negotiate outside the scope of personal constructs gives rise to anxiety.

ROGER'S SELF THEORY

Every person strives for fulfilment and tries to cultivate an 'ideal self'. Congruence between a person's perception of themselves and their ideal self is important. Individuals who attain and maintain this congruence are able to self-actualize, achieve and be successful in both psychological and social aspects of their personality. Anxiety stems from behaviour not in keeping with one's own self-image.

DEVELOPMENT OF FEARS

Fear is an unpleasant emotion in reaction to a perceived danger (imminent or ongoing). Infants are generally fearless and most fears are acquired/learnt (see Table 5.2).

Table 5.2 Development of fears

Age	Fears
Newborn	Visual cliff
6–12 months	Darkness; height
12 months–3 years	Strangers; separation
3–6 years	Learn fear responses; animals
6–12 years	Social shame
Teenage onwards	Failure; illness; death
Adulthood	Neurotic/stress-related disorders

Fears can be learned and maintained by both classical and operant conditioning. Some fears are more easily acquired (**stimulus preparedness**), perhaps because of an evolutionary genetic predisposition. Fears can also be developed and sustained by social learning and modelling.

LANGUAGE DEVELOPMENT

- *Language*: the requisite skills for communication
- *Phoneme*: unit of sound
- *Morpheme*: meaningful units of sound (e.g. words). Contain phonemes
- *Semantics*: meaning
- *Syntax*: grammar.

Table 5.3 Stages of language development

Age	Language development
3 months	Babbling (series of phonemes)
9 months	Repetitive babbling; imitate mother's speech acts
12 months	Speaks three words
18 months	Speaks any one of 18–40 words
24 months	Vocabulary >240 words; grammatically pairs words; telegraphic speech
36 months	Early comprehension of grammar and syntax
48 months	Correct use of grammar; language comprehension better than expression
60 months	Language akin to adult speech

The acquisition of language (see Table 5.3) and the learning of communication skills can be affected by a variety of factors. There is growing evidence through work done with feral children that the capacity to learn language is limited to early childhood.

Language is slower to develop in:

- *biological situations*
  - in boys
  - with intrauterine growth retardation
  - following a prolonged second stage of labour
  - in twins
  - with a lack of stimulation (e.g. hearing impairment)
- *environmental situations*
  - in large families
  - in those from social classes IV and V
  - with a lack of stimulation (e.g. neglect).

SEXUAL DEVELOPMENT

EMBRYOLOGY

Gonads initially appear as gonadal ridges (week 5). Primordial germ cells appear in gonadal ridges 1 week later (week 6). Gonads acquire morphological characteristics week 7. Sex is determined by the chromosomes carried by the germ cells: XY → male; XX → female.

Y chromosome carries testis-determining factor and results in gonads developing medullary cords (→ testes) and tunica albuginea, while suppressing the development of the cortical cords (→ ovaries).

The gonads then release hormones which influence further sex differentiation and the development of external genitalia.

Testes stimulate mesonephric ducts to form vas deferens and epididymis. Testicular androgens stimulate formation of penis, scrotum and prostate.

Ovaries stimulate paramesonephric ducts to form uterus, fallopian tubes and upper one-third of vagina. Oestrogen stimulates the formation of labia, clitoris and lower two-thirds of vagina.

Sexual identity: biological status as male/female.

Gender identity: person's self-awareness/perception as male/female. Usually achieved by age 5 years. Possible developmental theories:

- *Cognitive*: at less than 5 years understanding of gender is incomplete. Cognitive development increases self-awareness and after age 5 children have usually developed perception of their gender and associated role
- *Psychoanalytical*: Freud's theory of sexual development. Through repression and identification children acquire gender role having successfully negotiated Oedipal/ Electra complexes
- *Social learning*: children acquire self and gender identity through modelling and internalizing social and gender behaviours. However, attempts to raise baby boys with damaged/deficient genitalia as girls have generally failed.

    Usually gender and sexual identity correspond but in transsexuals they do not.

Gender role: masculine and feminine behaviours that correspond to gender, identifying individual as male/female (stems from cultural gender stereotypes).

Sex/gender typing: differential treatment of boys and girls. Influences acquisition of gender identity and gender role.

Sexual orientation/preference: preference regarding sexual partner. Heterosexual (opposite sex partner), homosexual (same sex partner) and bisexual (both).

Debate over whether innate (biological determinism) or learnt. Tentative findings concerning sexual orientation/preference:

- established prior to puberty and sexual activity
- parental interaction/influence and nature of initial sexual experiences are of little determining importance.

Sexual drive: basic need for sexual gratification.

ADOLESCENCE

PUBERTY

Changes associated with the development of reproductive ability.

Described as primary (concern sex organs) and secondary sexual changes:

- *Males*: average onset 11.5 years of age. Initially there is an increase in size of the testes and then the penis and the appearance of pubic hair. There is also a change of body proportions, an overall increase in size, the appearance of facial and body hair and a lowering of vocal pitch
- *Females*: average onset 11 years of age. Commences in most cases with breast development (thelarche) but in some (20 per cent) begins with pubic hair growth. First menses (menarche) occurs on average at 13–14 years of age.

CONFLICT

Conflict with authority is a feature often associated with puberty/adolescence. Culturally this view is more prevalent in Western societies.

Possible explanations for conflict during this period:

- *ethology*: conflict forces adolescent to adapt and forge role/identity/purpose
- *separation–individuation*: expectancy (societal) and desire (personal) for ongoing dependence (on authority/parents) conflict with ability to be socially independent
- *cognitive development*: intellectual maturation prompts desires that may differ from/ oppose traditional views
- *Erikson's psychosocial development*: adolescent seeks to create personal identity and achieve autonomy.

NB most adolescents undergo puberty without significant conflict.

AFFECTIVE STABILITY

There is a slight increase in emotional instability during adolescence. This is due to both psychosocial and biological changes that accompany this period. Significant adolescent affective instability tends to persist into adulthood.

ADAPTATIONS IN ADULT LIFE

Adaptation continues throughout life. Common adaptations include:

PAIRING

The development of a permanent romantic relationship has a positive effect on mental and physical health (i.e. stable fulfilling relationship is protective and promotes health).
   The selection of a suitable partner is influenced by several factors:

- *attitudes*: partners tend to come from similar cultural background and have similar socio-economic status
- *partners that offer best cost–benefit ratio* are preferred (social exchange theory)
- relationships in which both partners feel equity (in cost–benefit ratio) are preferred (equity theory)
- *attractiveness*: seek similar level of attractiveness even though would desire a more attractive person than oneself (matching hypothesis). Imbues sense of security as individual feels less likely to be rejected.

   Different cultures place differential emphasis on certain attributes. Men from most cultures rate physical attractiveness highly while women place greater emphasis on drive and economic success.

PARENTING

Parenthood affects both the parents and their relationship, which usually becomes more affectionate despite possible stresses (reduced income, sleep, personal space and time).
   Fathers and mothers adopt more 'feminine behaviours'.
   Good parenting (affectionate, caring and supportive) enhances child's self-esteem. Bad parenting (abuse, neglect) increases likelihood of later problems.

ILLNESS

Acute illness is a common stressor, prompting concern about socio-economic future. Likelihood of illness and coping strategies change with age. Chronic illness leads to adjustment in stages:

- *shock*: sense of disbelief
- *encounter*: react by grieving and possibly becoming depressed

- *retreat*: use denial to avoid dealing with illness or its consequences
- *intrusion*: gradual adaptation and acceptance of fate.

GRIEF, BEREAVEMENT AND LOSS

GRIEF

The affective, behavioural and cognitive concomitants of bereavement. Typical grief involves (cf. illness):

- initial sense of disbelief and shock
- emotional arousal as loss becomes apparent
- denial of anger
- biological symptoms of depression, e.g. sleep disturbance, changes of appetite and weight
- identification with deceased.

BEREAVEMENT

The process following the death of a loved person.
Stages of bereavement:

Protest: initially in a state of shock: stunned and feeling numbed, denial
Preoccupation: involves yearning for subject of loss – illusions and hallucinations; some symptoms of depression
Disorganization: disruption of routine, irritability
Resolution: eventually come to terms with loss; accept and adjust to reality.

NB bereaved more likely to consult their family doctor and at increased risk of dying during first 6 months.
Predictors of poor resolution or adjustment:

- loss of child/spouse
- loss is unexpected
- occurs at time of additional stresses
- from poorer socio-economic background
- ambivalent/dependent relationship with deceased.

Typically grief resolves within 6–12 months.

MOURNING

The voluntary social/cultural expression of loss.

AGEING

Ageing brings about certain characteristic changes, often described as losses.

FUNCTIONAL

Physiological functions decline at varying rates: notably – vision, hearing, new learning, decision making. However, some cognitive functions may improve (e.g. memory) through practice or experience.

PSYCHOSOCIAL

Psychosocial changes are less predictable. Stigma attached to ageing (particularly in Western societies). More likely to be lonely. Social isolation (sensory decline/deficits → less likely to socialize; fewer friends). Sexual drive and enjoyment may remain intact but socially not accepted. Individuals become less neurotic and more able to contain emotionality.

DEATH AND DYING

The realization of imminent or impending death may lead to the following phases (after Kübler-Ross):

- *denial*: disbelief; refusal to accept reality; reject diagnosis
- *anger*: 'why me'; blaming
- *bargaining*: attempt to negotiate a better outcome
- *depression*: outpouring of feelings; may become clinically depressed
- *acceptance*: resolution of above phases; calm and understanding.

It is increasingly recognized that these phases do not necessarily resolve in rigid sequence.

Adjustment to death involves both the dying individual and their family and friends. Communication and compassion help both the patient and those around them to adapt.

Social sciences

6

DEFINITIONS

SOCIAL CLASS

A population sub-group defined by relatively stable social parameters:

*M*oney (financial wealth)
*O*ccupation
type of *R*esidence and its location
*E*ducational achievement.

Essentially, the MORE you have the higher your **socio-economic status**. Unlike some other social systems (e.g. the Hindu caste system), there is potential mobility (up or down) between classes through educational and financial means.

The Registrar-General's classification (introduced 1911) divides society into six hierarchical social classes. In Britain, social class is primarily based on occupation and decided according to the head of a household. The social classes are labelled O, V, IV, III, II and I: unemployed, unskilled, semi-skilled, skilled, intermediate and professional, respectively.

PSYCHIATRIC DISORDER AND SOCIAL CLASS

Socio-economic status is a very strong predictor of morbidity and the relationship extends to psychiatric disorders. The reasons for this may be:

- *social causation theory*: the greater environmental stress and adversity experienced by the lower social classes in some way contributes to the development of psychological ill-health;
- *social selection/drift theory*: those with psychiatric illness are not equipped to remain in the higher social classes and so either remain in the lower social classes or gravitate towards them;

- *differential treatment/labelling*: race and social class bias the management of those with psychiatric illnesses, producing a misrepresentation in the lower classes.

Psychiatric disorders more commonly diagnosed in lower social classes:

- alcohol dependence
- schizophrenia
- depression
- illicit drug abuse
- psychopathy.

Those more commonly found in higher social classes:

- bipolar affective disorder
- eating disorders.

SOCIAL CLASS AND PSYCHIATRIC HEALTHCARE

The utilization of psychiatric healthcare services has been described by Goldberg and Huxley as a series of five levels. Movement from one level to the next entails successfully negotiating through a filter:

- *Level I*: The community
  - *Filter 1*: Illness behaviour prompting decision to seek help
- *Level II*: GP attenders
  - *Filter 2*: Detection of disorder by GP
- *Level III*: Diagnosed as ill
  - *Filter 3*: Decision as to whether specialist help is needed
- *Level IV*: Specialist service attendees
  - *Filter 4*: Decision to hospitalize
- *Level V*: Specialist service inpatient.

Decisions as to when and how individuals move through a healthcare system are based on:

- *characteristics of the service*: funding, waiting lists, geographical convenience etc.
- *nature of the disorder*: severity, risk to patient and others etc.
- *social aspects of the individual*: age, gender, race, status etc.

Psychiatric patients from poorer socio-economic backgrounds are more likely to:

- become psychiatric inpatients
- remain as inpatients for longer periods of time
- be subjected to physical treatments such as electro-convulsive therapy (ECT).

These health inequalities were highlighted by the 1980 **Black Report** which examined health in relation to social class. It reported that, in comparison with those from social class I, individuals from social class V:

- have double the neonatal mortality
- are twice as likely to die prior to retirement
- have an increased incidence of most diseases.

Reasons proposed for these inequalities are:

- good health promotes an improvement in social class and vice versa
- economic power determines ability to 'purchase' good health; e.g. better food, residence and lifestyle
- disease-promoting behaviours are more strongly associated with the lower social classes, e.g. smoking.

THE DOCTOR–PATIENT RELATIONSHIP

DOCTOR'S ROLE

An individual's expected pattern of social behaviour is their **social role**. For doctors and patients **Parsons** put forward a model incorporating their rights and obligations.
A doctor's social role is to:

- diagnose and define illness
- offer support and treatment
- legitimize illness and patient sick role.

Doctors therefore confer the **sick role**, which gives the patient certain rights and obligations:

- *rights*: exempt from blame, i.e. not responsible for having illness; excused from usual/normal duties, e.g. household activities or work.
- *obligations*: to desire recovery and to seek necessary help; to cooperate in the assessment and management of their illness.

ILLNESS BEHAVIOUR

Mechanic defined illness behaviour as 'the ways in which given symptoms may be differentially perceived, evaluated and acted upon'.
Abnormal illness behaviour has been defined by **Pilowsky** as 'the persistence of a maladaptive mode of experiencing, perceiving, evaluating and responding to one's own health status'. The illness behaviour is disproportionate to the underlying disease (real or not).
There is a tendency among doctors caring for those with abnormal illness behaviour to focus on somatic symptoms, often leading to inappropriate treatment which may inadvertently reinforce the abnormal behaviour (e.g. somatization disorders).

PSYCHIATRIC DISORDERS AND FAMILIES

There are important interactions between some of the major mental illnesses and aspects of family life.

SCHIZOPHRENIA

Theories originally thought to explain the aetiology of schizophrenia:

- Disordered communication: *double-bind (Bateson)* Abnormal parental communication during childhood generates ambivalence. Messages conflicting, incompatible and vague, causing confusion and ambiguity. Child receives 'contradictory injunctions' from which there is no satisfactory escape. Formerly thought to precipitate withdrawal, irrational behaviour and eventually schizophrenia. *Wynne and Singer* suggested that abnormal family communication (non-sequential, disrupted) led to schizophrenia in offspring.
- Abnormal (deviant) role relationships: *Schizophrenogenic mother (Fromm–Reichman)*. Specific maternal characteristics lead to schizophrenia in offspring: **HORrID**
  Hostile
  Overprotective
  Rejecting
  Indifferent
  Distant.
- *Marital schism/skew (Lidz)*: schism – parental division because of conflict splits child's loyalties. Skew – dominant, intrusive mother and submissive, compliant father leads to maternal eccentricities dominating family and intruding into child's life causing disturbance.
- *Expressed emotion (Vaughn and Leff)*: expressed emotion (EE) >35 hours per week better predictor of relapse than compliance with medication. EE characterized by critical comments, hostility and emotional over-involvement. In certain centres family therapy has been shown to be as effective as antipsychotics in relapse prevention.

ALCOHOL ABUSE AND DEPENDENCE

Drinking excessively leads to a variety of problems (violence, psychological distress/disorders, the abuse of other substances, financial loss). These have a detrimental effect on family relationships.

Around half of all alcohol abusers have an associated psychiatric disorder. The commonest are: antisocial personality disorder > mania > schizophrenia > major depression.

DEPRESSION

Early research (Brown and Harris) identified certain vulnerability factors relating to women: maternal loss before 11 years of age, having three or more children below the age of 15 years, lack of employment outside the home and the lack of a confidante.

LIFE EVENTS

Life events (LEs see page 12) have major implications and produce lasting change (technically a LE can be positive or negative but in a psychiatric context the latter is usually implied).

LEs can be assessed by Holmes and Rahe Social Readjustment Rating Scale (self-report questionnaire) or Life Events and Difficulties Schedule (LEDS). Latter is a more reliable and valid measure which entails a semi-structured interview.

Schizophrenia: LEs significant in terms of relapse and course of illness but not onset.

Depression: severe abuse (violent, sexual, emotional) during childhood is related to development of depression. LEs four times more likely to have occurred in year prior to depressive illness compared to those without depression. Losses (material and psychological) are of particular importance, leading to feelings of low self-esteem, humiliation, hopelessness and entrapment. Suicide attempts are highly anticipated by significant LEs.

Puerperal psychosis: studies show little relationship with LEs, particularly in patients with previous psychotic illness.

Mania: association with LEs unclear. However, viewed as a manifestation of manic defences, mania may be a reactionary event.

INSTITUTIONS

Generally contain a selected population. They have rules and routines, which can lead to problems of under-stimulation, isolation and loss of independence, skills and status. Institutionalization can thus lead to diminished motivation, apathy and social withdrawal.

Social institutions are those in which members have agreed forms of relationship (e.g. families). **Total institutions** isolate people from the outside world for a considerable length of time under a highly regulated regime (e.g. prisons, traditional psychiatric hospitals).

Goffman (1961) highlighted the disadvantages of total institutions such as large psychiatric hospitals and described institutionalization and institutional life:

* *binary living and binary management*: staff appear to live in a different world to that of the patients they manage;
* *batch living*: the normal components of life (working, home life and leisure) are often absent in institutions;
* *mortification process*: the process of becoming an inhabitant of a total institution. It begins with the **betrayal funnel** (relatives send the patient to hospital with the help of health professionals) and involves **role-stripping** (admission to hospital – removal of personal effects, 'stripping' for physical examination, bathing and being given new clothes) and adoption of **patient role**.

He also described the reactions of patients to this process: rebellion, withdrawal, pretence to compliance (colonization), conversion, institutionalization.

Many of those who showed withdrawal had additional symptoms (submissiveness, apathy, diminished self-esteem and an inability to plan) that Barton grouped under the syndrome of **institutional neurosis**.

The Three Mental Hospitals Study (Netherne, Mapperley, Severals) found that the extent of clinical poverty (poverty of speech, social withdrawal, blunted affect) in schizophrenic patients was associated with the poverty of their social environment.

Important theorists and their concepts

7

SIGMUND FREUD (1856–1939)

Regarded as the founder of **psychoanalysis**: a conversation with a psychotherapist intended to help the subject acquire insights about their unconscious. Freud did not invent psychoanalysis but brought together the various elements and developed and popularized them. Originally a neuroanatomist, he came to psychoanalysis in his forties.

Inspired by:

- Charcot (initial work on hysteria and hypnosis strongly affected Freud)
- Brucke (concepts of conservation and energy)
- Meynert (linked neuroanatomy to behavioural consequences)
- Helmholz (distribution of energy, modelling psychological theories upon physical ones)
- Hughlings Jackson (from whom theories relating to association and regression, and release phenomena, are derived).

Selected publications:

- *The Neuro-Psychoses of Defence* (1894)
- *Studies on Hysteria* (1895, with Bruer): early work, influenced by Charcot
- *Project for a Scientific Psychology*: associated with 'nirvana'; the tendency to minimise arousal
- *The Interpretation of Dreams* (1900)
- *Psychobiology of Everyday Life* (1901): introduced idea of the 'Freudian slip' (not his term); a verbal parapraxis that reveals an unconscious thought
- *Three Essays on the Theory of Sexuality* (1905): psychosexual development
- *Totem and Taboo* (1913): explored incest
- *Mourning and Melancholia* (1917): explored parallels between bereavement and depression in terms of loss
- *Group Psychology and the Analysis of the Ego* (1921): crowd behaviour, groups/ leaders

- *The Ego and the Id* (1923)
- *Civilization and its Discontents* (1930): expressed the view that Man is trapped between his instincts and cultural norms.

TOPOGRAPHICAL MODEL

Freud's first model concerning levels of Mind; described in *The Interpretation of Dreams*:

1 **Conscious**: Awareness of external and internal perceptions:
   - involves **secondary process thinking** (see Table 7.1)
   - governed by the **reality principle** (involves delayed gratification and is the result of external reality)
   - content is readily accessible
2 **Pre-conscious**: Holds information which person may be unaware of at any particular moment but can call up at will if necessary through selective attention, e.g. the layout of their house, colour of their car etc.
   Develops during childhood (parallel to the development of the Ego). Like the conscious Mind, involves secondary process thinking and is governed by reality principle
3 **Unconscious**: All mental processes outside of consciousness. Repressed ideas, memories, feelings and urges:
   - entails **primary process** thinking (see Table 7.1)
   - governed by the **pleasure principle** (largely innate and involves seeking pleasure and avoiding pain; the immediate gratification of instinctual drives leading to wish fulfilment)
   - information is only accessible when pre-conscious is bypassed or compromised, e.g. dreaming, drugs/alcohol, hypnosis, psychological stress.

Table 7.1 Primary and secondary process thinking

	Primary process thinking	Secondary process thinking
Time	Timelessness	Linear forward flow of time
Organization	Lacking	Systematized
Reality	Disregard of conscious world reality	Regard for external reality
Logical connections	Disregarded	Regarded and respected
Contradictions	Not recognized	Acknowledged but not always accepted
Tolerance for inconsistency	High	Low
Governing principle	Pleasure	Reality

STRUCTURAL MODEL

Described in *The Ego and the Id*; superseded the topographical model.

1 **Id**: entirely unconscious reserve of impulses, drives, instincts. These basic drives concerning aggression, survival, sex etc. influence thinking (primary process) in accordance with the pleasure principle. It is non-verbal, illogical and has the following components:
   - *eros*: life instinct, creative force
   - *thanatos*: death instinct, destructive and aggressive elements

– *libido*: derived from the Id, manifests initially as Ego libido (primary narcissism) and then object libido
2 **Ego**: the Ego is the integrator; that part of the personality that mediates with the external world. Fulfils its executive function through negotiating the demands of the Id, the Super-Ego and external reality. Functions at conscious, preconscious and unconscious levels, adapting through use of *defences*. The *Ego-ideal* is what the individual aspires to (mental parental images)
3 **Super-Ego**: the censor of the personality; an individual's morals, values and ethics as derived from their parents (tells an individual what not to do). Conscious component is termed conscience (individual is aware of their morality but not the processes that generate or sustain it). Develops in the second year of life, established by 5 years.

PSYCHOTHERAPY AND THE PSYCHOTHERAPEUTIC RELATIONSHIP

Freud initially used **hypnosis** to help manifest suppressed thoughts. However, it was often unsuccessful and he came to believe it hindered the free flow of thought. He therefore developed the **concentration method**, which required the patient to lie down, close their eyes and concentrate on their symptoms. Freud would facilitate the process by the use of leading questions and by placing his hands on the patient's forehead. This was used to recall memories associated with the symptoms. Freud then progressed to **free association** in which again the patient is lying down but with open eyes. The patient is then asked to voice any and all their thoughts as they arise, without reservation or censorship.

Central to psychotherapy are the concepts of **therapeutic alliance** (mutual cooperation), **transference** [the unconscious displacement of significant past relationships (usually relatives) onto the therapist by the patient] and **counter-transference** (the conscious feelings, emotions and attitudes of the therapist towards the patient). It is by working with and through these processes that 'psychotherapy' is achieved. **Resistance** is obstruction/reluctance by the patient to access their unconscious.

PSYCHOSEXUAL DEVELOPMENT

Freud proposed that psychosexual development took place in stages (NB ages double, i.e. 1½, 3, 6 and 12 years):

PRE-GENITAL PHASE

- 0–18 months   **Oral phase**: pleasure is derived from oral activity and there is a preoccupation with feeding.
  Sucking stage: passive early oral (receptive) phase.
  Biting stage: aggressive oral (sadistic) phase
- 18–36 months   **Anal phase**: Attention is focused on excretory processes. Infant has to adapt to the demands of others.
  Expulsive and retentive phases
- 3–6 years   **Phallic phase**: increasing focus on genitalia; libido directed towards others.

Involves castration anxiety, penis envy, Oedipal* complex in males and Electra† complex in females (attachment to opposite-sex parent and aggression towards same-sex parent)

- 6–12 years   **Latency**: lasts until onset of puberty. Involves the recognition, acknowledgement and acceptance of reality.

*Oedipal complex: in Sophocles' tragedy Oedipus Rex kills his father and marries his mother, not knowing their true identities. †Electra complex: from Greek mythology – Electra plans the death of her mother Clytemnestra, responsible for the murder of her father.

GENITAL PHASE

- 12 years–adult   Acquisition of sexual maturity (homosexual and heterosexual experiences). Increasing identification with same-sex parent.

DREAMS

Freud described dreams as the 'royal road to the unconscious'. He set out the composition of dreams and certain principles for their interpretation:

- dreams aim to preserve sleep
- they consist of **latent** and **manifest** components
- dreams represent the fulfilment of **unconscious wishes**.

Latent component (i.e. underlying message) is disguised and transformed into the manifest component (the apparently bizarre content) through dream work which consists of four mechanisms:

- *dramatization/symbolization*: symbols are used to represent abstract ideas
- *displacement*: latent content is replaced by obscurely related elements
- *condensation*: latent elements are fused and abbreviated
- *secondary elaboration*: the revision that occurs upon waking; rationalizing the dream.

ANNA FREUD (1892–1982)

Daughter of Sigmund Freud. Important figure in the development of child analysis. Along with others, further developed the theory of **defence mechanisms** (first introduced by her father): the unconscious filters and modifiers of unacceptable thoughts/aspects of oneself.

Defences are generally a normal, healthy aspect of psychological functioning and can be categorized as narcissistic, neurotic, primitive/higher, immature/mature.

CUPIDS RAFT
Compensation: attempts (conscious/unconscious) to make up for perceived deficiencies within oneself.
Conversion: physical symptoms produced by unconscious psychological distress (formerly termed hysteria).

Undoing*: (symbolic atonement) the neutralisation of unacceptable behaviour by some counteract. Similar to reaction formation.

Projection*: psychological aspects of oneself deemed unacceptable are disowned and incorporated into another person.

Projective identification: the identification with projected aspects of oneself.

Intellectualization: closely related to rationalization; the use of intellectual concepts and processes to avoid emotional expression. Affective experiences are thought about rather than experienced.

Isolation*: the separation of a thought from its associated affect.

Idealization: overestimation of an object's qualities.

Introjection*: the transposition of external objects and their qualities into the self; the symbolic assimilation and internalization of an object. Central to the development of the Ego and Super-Ego, it is a form of identification and the 'opposite' of projection.

Identification: unconscious adoption of the attributes of others, influencing the individual's self-esteem through association. Important in the development of the Super-Ego.

Incorporation: thought to commence in the oral phase, this is a special form of introjection that is central to the process of identification. It is a primitive defence that involves the acquisition of another individual's characteristics (typically the parent's).

Denial: lack of awareness for an objective reality.

Displacement: the redirection of attitudes/drives from their primary object to a more acceptable/less threatening substitute.

Distortion: the remodelling and alteration of external reality to meet personal requirements or wishes.

Dissociation: detachment of particular mental processes from others. This psychological separation leads to compartmentalization of functioning.

Suppression: the voluntary (and so not considered to be a true defence by some) sanctioning of unacceptable ideas from the conscious. The underlying impulse/conflict can be recalled.

Sublimation*: the diversion of socially unacceptable instincts and drives into socially appropriate activities.

Substitution: a highly valued but unachievable goal or object is unconsciously supplanted by one more easily realized.

Symbolization: representation of objectionable ideas/objects with neutral ones through unconscious means. Results in the transfer/displacement of associated emotions to the symbol.

Splitting: an inability to integrate opposing aspects of personality. Manifests as the polarized division of objects into good or bad.

Repression*: most basic defence (originally described by Freud) and most commonly employed. Unacceptable ideas, impulses or feelings are banished to the unconscious.

Regression*: retreat to a maturationally earlier level of functioning. Lower level of complexity makes gratification more attainable.

Reaction formation*: subject reacts against unacceptable impulses by superimposing an opposing behaviour or attitude. It involves two steps: the repression of an unacceptable thought followed by the expression of its direct opposite.

Rationalization: retrospective justification by rational/logical/acceptable means for ideas, feelings or behaviours that actually have different, unconscious motives. Differs from lying, which is a conscious process.

Reversal*: an instinct which, though maintaining its aim, is reversed in its choice of object.

Restitution: replacement of a lost, highly valued object by another.

Acting out: behavioural expression of unconscious emotional difficulties without being aware of its significance.

Fixation: (on a person/object) excessive gratification at an immature level of development because of arrested maturation.

Fantasy: daydreaming; the creation of mental imagery for events. Often an escape from reality that allows the fulfilment of wishes.

Turning against the self*: an example of displacement in which impulses directed at others (e.g. aggression) are turned against oneself.

*associated with Anna Freud.

CARL GUSTAV JUNG (1875–1961)

Born in Kesswil, Switzerland; only child until the age of 9. Member of Freud's group and influenced by works of Immanuel Kant, Friedrich Nietzsche, Emmanuel Swedenborg and Richard von Kraft-Ebing. Broke away in early 1900s to found **Analytical Psychology**.

Causality: Explanation in terms of the past.

Teleology: Explanation in terms of future potential.

Synchronicity: Explanation in terms of the interface between the physical and mystic world.

Levels of psyche: Personal unconscious (relatively superficial and accessible), **collective unconscious** (also called the objective psyche – universal memories/primordial images of mankind, containing inherited cultural and racial elements; gives rise to consciousness) and conscious (includes **persona**).

Libido: Jungian theory places less emphasis on the sexual role of the libido; instead libido stems from all psychic energy, which has two basic *attitudes*. **Introversion** is an inwardly directed libido manifest as self-preoccupation, and **extroversion** is an outwardly directed libido. Jung did however retain the concept of Ego.

Psychological functions: Four basic operations of the Mind (*FIST*):

Feelings
Intuition
Sensations
Thinking.

Combination of the two attitudes (introversion/extroversion) and four functions creates eight psychological types (e.g. extrovert feeling, introvert feeling and so on).

Attitude Type + Functional Type → Psychological Type.

ARCHETYPES

Prototypes of figures manifest in the collective unconscious through archetypal images, featuring in dreams and myths, as an expression of man's psychological nature.

- *Persona* (mask portraying mood in Greek drama): 'social mask' enveloping the personality. Allows individual to conform to social expectation whilst maintaining personal needs. That part of consciousness that interacts and negotiates with external reality.
- *Soul-image* (anima and animus): the unconscious aspect of persona. **Animus**, male prototypical archetype; the male component of female personality. **Anima**, female prototypical archetype; the female component of male personality.
- *Shadow*: unconscious aspect of the Ego, comprising repressed/primitive animal instincts (i.e. unacknowledged aspects of self).
- *Others*: Wise Old Man, Great Mother, Hero.

Archetype + Experience (i.e. interaction with the world) → Complexes (networks of ideas and thoughts linked through commonality of emotions and feelings).

INDIVIDUATION

Growth of an individual's personality leading to self-realization and understanding. A basic function of the Ego.

SELF

Develops as individual deals with other archetypes, binding together conscious and unconscious elements. The goal of individuation; a complete, whole personality.
   Jung's ideas have been criticized for being too mystical and difficult to test.

MELANIE KLEIN (1882–1960)

Born in Vienna, the youngest of four. Became an important figure in the British Psycho-Analytical Society (founded by Ernest Jones). One of the key developers of child analysis (along with Anna Freud), advocating the use of play as a means of gaining insight into a child's psychological world.
   Basic Ego functions first described by Klein include integration and synthesis. Placed more emphasis on the role of the mother in psychosexual development of children than Freud had done, believing that Oedipal-type conflicts occurred much earlier than postulated by Freud.
   Placed less emphasis on the actual experiences of the infant and more on its internal, fantasy world.

OBJECT-RELATIONS THEORY

Personality development is linked to the internalization of experiences/relationships (objects) from the external world. Though not commonly regarded as an object-relations theorist, Klein was one of the first to discuss this phenomenon.

PARANOID–SCHIZOID POSITION

Develops in first few months of life and features sense of persecution and isolation (Ego is also thought to develop during this time). Infant uses primitive defences of **splitting, projection** and **introjection** in dealing with the world and its environment. Death instinct (Freud) leads to destructive rage. Frustration and anxiety are seen as necessary for the development and growth of the infant's personality. Good objects are internalized (introjected) whilst bad objects are projected.

DEPRESSIVE POSITION

Commences as infant begins to recognize its mother (aged 6 months) and become aware of the imperfections of the world. Comes to view objects as a whole; reconciles good and bad component of mother as one (is able to both love and hate her). Anxiety is transformed from paranoid to depressive form. Recognizes it is separate from mother and attributes this to its **aggression** (and regrets this). Linked to manic defences.

ALFRED ADLER (1870–1937)

Viennese doctor, associate of Freud but broke away (placed a greater emphasis on social factors than on instinct) to form school of **individual psychology**: each individual achieves their particular personal goals in their own unique manner. A key influence in the development of day hospitals and therapeutic groups, though he himself did not go on to explore/develop these concepts.

ORGAN INFERIORITY

Individuals have a desire for superiority through self-improvement, and seek a particular lifestyle. This relates to their need for others and a desire for a sense of belonging. At birth the individual starts in an inferior position which causes anxiety and so the individual attempts to overcome this.

The conscious and unconscious conflict that drives an individual to strive to overcome their anxiety is described as their **inferiority complex** (particularly when their desire or attempts at self-improvement are blocked or fail). Neuroses are then dysfunctional means by which individuals deal with their perceived inferiority. Described **masculine protest** as women's attempt to escape their perceived submissive, inferior role.

In Adlerian theory individuals are able to direct their fate as opposed to being subject to unconscious drives. Creativity and social cooperation are essential primary qualities of human beings.

AARON T. BECK (1921–)

A key figure in the development of cognitive therapy, and particularly in the development of the **cognitive model of depression**. Noticed that most depressed people had similar/recurrent thinking. Focused on the importance of these cognitions in the generation and maintenance of psychopathology (i.e. the experience is less important than the interpretation).

Suggested that negative cognitions beget depression, rather than the other way around. Latent dysfunctional beliefs (or negative core beliefs/**cognitive schemas**), e.g. everyone should like me, are activated by an environmental trigger (stress-diathesis model), e.g. a rejection, and precipitate a lowering of mood. If the subject then becomes depressed, this is maintained by negative automatic thinking (NAT).

NAT relates to self, the world and the future (the **cognitive triad**). Although Beck appears not to have specifically included the past, this is an important aspect of NAT. These thoughts are based on **cognitive distortions**: *arbitrary inference* (drawing ill-founded conclusions), *selective abstraction* (only focusing on one aspect of an experience), *overgeneralization* (drawing conclusions based on a single event), *minimization/maximization* (underestimating the significance of a positive event, and vice versa), *personalization* (taking things personally) and *dichotomous thinking* ('all-or-nothing', i.e. there are no shades of experience, only entirely good or entirely bad).

ADOLF MEYER (1866–1950)

Founded **psychobiology**. Comprehensive and pluralistic approach to understanding psychological illnesses. Brought together biological and psychosocial aspects; **holistic approach**.

Aimed to understand people and their illnesses in simplest possible terms (common-sense psychiatry).

KAREN HORNEY (1885–1952)

A Neo-Feudian (along with Sullivan, Fromm and Erikson) who emphasized the importance of social influences on the development of self through interpersonal interactions.

Developed **holistic psychology**. Stressed the principle of **basic anxiety**.

Child could cope with the environment by moving:

- *towards* people: compliant person
- *against* people: aggressive person
- *away* from people: detached person.

Horney's concept of the self:

- *actual self*
- *real self*
- *idealized self.*

Therapy involved: self-actualization, self-realization and dealing with the here and now.

HARRY STACK SULLIVAN (1892–1949)

A Neo-Freudian. Helped develop **interpersonal psychotherapy** (IPT), which stems from the idea that interpersonal experiences form the basis of personality development through **reflected appraisal** and **consensual evaluation**.

Typically used as a brief intervention in depression, IPT focuses on the patient's relationships in four main areas: grief (associated with loss), disputes (with significant others), deficit (in social interaction) and role transition (negotiating the phases of life, e.g. getting married, becoming a parent, changing career etc.).

DONALD WINNICOTT (1897–1971)

An object-relations theorist (along with Balint, Guntrip and Fairburn): views the internalization of early relationships (e.g. with parents) as integral to personality development. Initially trained as a paediatrician, went on to study the early mother–baby relationship:

- *Good-enough mother*: responsive to baby's needs, adequately meeting these by balancing frustration and gratification. Through good parenting, child gains autonomy and develops capacity to be alone.
- *Pathological mother*: gives personal needs priority. Baby creates a **false self** so as to protect **true self**.
- *Transitional objects/space*: between ages of 4 and 18 months infant uses an object (e.g. 'comfort blanket') to help allay anxiety aroused by process of separation-individuation (i.e. from relating with the internal world to relating with the external world). These objects represent both the self and the mother.

KARL ABRAHAM (1877–1925)

Student of Sigmund Freud. Expanded upon Freud's psychosexual stages of development. Subdivided some stages further:

- oral stage → sucking and biting phases (receptive/sadistic respectively)
- anal stage → anal–sadistic (destructive–expulsive) and anal–erotic (mastering-retentive) phases.

GORDON ALLPORT (1897–1967)

Founder of **humanistic** school of psychology. Individual strives to develop self-identity. Selfhood is achieved in stages.

ERIC BERNE (1910–1970)

Helped develop **transactional analysis**, which focuses on restoring self-esteem by 'strokes' (positive responses) and 'injunctions' (negative responses) in short-term group sessions.

Described individuals as having three **Ego states** (cf. Freud's Id, Ego and Super-Ego): **Child** (childhood primitive elements); **Adult** (component that is able to appraise reality objectively); **Parent** (represents the values/ideals of the individual). Used the term **games** to describe the interaction between these Ego states.

WILFRED BION (1897–1979)

Applied the ideas of psychoanalysis in a social context and described three **basic assumptions** (ways of being) which come up in group situations: pairing, fight–flight and dependency. These are automatic reactions that interfere with the functioning of the group, and are more powerfully present in autocratic situations where there may be little scope for open dialogue (e.g. business meetings, certain institutions etc). Emphasized analysis of the group.

S. H. FOULKES (1898–1976)

Born S. H. Fuchs in Germany where he trained in medicine, went on to become an important figure in British group, family and couple therapy. Helped formulate small group therapy based on his work in the Northfields Experiments, conducted in post-WWII Birmingham. Emphasized analysis of the group by the group, with the therapist facilitating individuals towards greater initiative and responsibility.

Regarded individuals as **nodes** within a network of relationships, and illness as a disturbance in that network. Illness could not therefore be adequately addressed by focusing exclusively on the individual. Argued that groups operated at several levels of psyche, ranging from the conscious (e.g. current adult relationships) to the unconscious (e.g. archetypal images, similar to Jung's ideas).

IRVIN D. YALOM (1931–)

Described certain therapeutic (curative) factors of groups (1995):

- *Universality*: recognition and sharing of common experiences
- *Altruism*: individuals think more about others and less about themselves, enabling them to develop their therapeutic strengths
- *Corrective recapitulation of the family group*: perceived problems in an individual's family background are re-enacted and addressed through the group
- *Imitative behaviour*: different models of behaviour, as demonstrated by the various individuals in the group, may be adopted by other individuals within the group

- *Interpersonal learning*: learning how an individual relates to the group and to other individuals within the group, and applying this to the wider social context
- *Cohesiveness*: sense of belonging, of being in an alliance
- *Existential factors*: recognition of the responsibility that comes with individuality, i.e. being responsible for who we are.
- *Others*: catharsis, insight, development of socialising techniques, instillation of hope, guidance.

SUMMARY OF OTHER IMPORTANT FIGURES

Table 7.2 Major contributions to psychotherapy and psychology

Important figure	Contributions to psychotherapy and psychology
RANK (1884–1939)	Anxiety stems from birth trauma. Primal anxiety
FERENCZI (1873–1933)	Active therapy and forced fantasies
ROGERS (1902–1987)	Client-centred psychotherapy, unconditional positive regard
KOHUT (1913–1981)	Founded school of self-psychology
MORENO (1889–1974)	Psychodrama
PERLS (1893–1970)	Gestalt therapy
REICH (1897–1951)	Character defences 'armour'. Character types: hysterical, narcissistic, masochistic, compulsive
RADO (1890–1972)	Adaptational psychodynamics
FROMM (1900–1980)	Types of personality: marketing, hoarding, receptive, exploitative, productive
MASLOW (1908–1970)	Self-actualization

Table 7.3 Important developments in therapy

Important figure	Therapy/treatment developed
FRANKL	Existential logotherapy
ELLIS	Rational Emotive Therapy
JANOV	Primal Therapy
ASSAGIOLI	Psychosynthesis
WOLPE	Systematic Desensitization
MONIZ	Psychosurgery
SAKEL	Insulin Coma Therapy
CHARPENTIER	Chlorpromazine
CADE	Lithium
KUHN	Imipramine
CERLETTI and BINI	Electroconvulsive Therapy (ECT)

Table 7.4 Noted associations of some important figures

Important figure	Noted association
BEARD	Neurasthenia
BRIQUET	Hysteria
BRAID	Neurohypnotism
CHARCOT	Hysteria/hypnosis
CULLEN	Neurosis
DURKHEIM	Anomie
ESQUIROL	Hallucinations
FALRET	La folie circulaire
GREISINGER	Neuropsychiatry
HECKER	Hebephrenia
HULL	Hypnosis
JANET	Hysteria/psychasthenia
MAXWELL	Therapeutic community
KAHLBAUM	Catatonia
LANGFELDT	Schizophreniform psychosis
MAY	Anxiety
MESMER	Hypnosis (animal magnetism)
MOREL	Demence precoce
SCHNEIDER	First rank symptoms
SHELDON	Body types
STAHL	Animism
SZASZ	Myth of mental illness
WATSON	Behaviourism

Psychopathology

Psychopathology concerns abnormalities of mind (states, processes, experience). It can be studied from experimental (biological), experiential (phenomenological) or explanatory (psychological) perspectives. Individual symptoms are rarely diagnostic; it is usually the pattern of symptoms (together with altered behaviour) that provides the basis for diagnosis.

Primary symptoms arise *de novo* and are the first (subjective) hallmarks of illness, whereas secondary symptoms can be attributed to another symptom or diagnosis (e.g. obsessional ideas in the context of depression).

Signs are recognized features of particular illnesses. The patient may not necessarily be aware of or mention them (e.g. flight of ideas in mania), and they can precede symptoms.

Phenomenology is a branch of medical nomenclature used in descriptive psychopathology. It is derived from observation and an empathic understanding of abnormal subjective experience.

NEUROSIS

Neurosis is a slightly outmoded 'catch-all' term encompassing psychopathology (symptoms/signs/diagnoses etc.) that cannot be directly attributed to an organic, psychotic, personality or developmental disorder. The ICD-10 is an excellent reference on neurotic symptomatology.

- *Compulsion*: obsessional impulses (imagined acts), e.g. to throw one's baby out of the pram or stab a pencil in one's eye. Distressing but rarely acted upon.
- *Conversion*: the manifestation of unconscious psychological distress as physical symptoms, i.e. the distress is somehow converted into physical form. **Dissociation** (formerly hysteria) is a form of conversion.
- *Dissociation*: separation of any aspect(s) of normal subjective experience (perceptions, emotions, motor control etc.) from conscious awareness as a result of psychological distress. Typically, the term is restricted to non-psychotic/organic/toxic states where the individual appears awake but manifests an impaired or distorted interaction with their surroundings relative to their pre-morbid state. Can be partial (as in dissociative amnesia or blindness) or complete (as in dissociative stupor).

- *Hypochondriasis*: subjects have the ill-founded (i.e. unreasonable) belief that they have a specific physical illness or abnormality. May be an over-valued idea or delusional fixity.
- *Obsession*: needlessly recurrent + pervasive + intrusive thought (*rumination*)/image/impulse (*compulsion*), recognized by the subject as their own, that is distressing and unwanted. Insight into the irrationality of obsessions distinguishes them from over-valued ideas.

  If a specific act/ritual is repeatedly/meticulously executed secondary to an obsessional fear (e.g. of contamination) in order to avert the imagined danger, this is termed an obsessive–compulsive symptom.
- *Phobia*: a quantitatively or (more rarely) qualitatively irrational fear of an object or situation that is both extreme and uncontrollable, sometimes despite appropriate insight.

  Note that phobic anxiety is activated by specific external cues; the associated thoughts/concerns are largely secondary to (i.e. based on) the fear. The opposite is true of obsessional disorders (i.e. the anxiety is based on the thoughts).
- *Rumination*: obsessional thoughts/thinking.
- *Somatization*: the complaint of a physical symptom (or symptoms) in the absence of any satisfactory physical explanation.

PHENOMENOLOGY OF THINKING/SPEECH

Our only insight into any thought disorder is the resultant disorder of language. Hence, the relevant nomenclature often refers to speech abnormalities and is sometimes vague and overlapping because it has evolved from descriptions by psychiatrists rather than systematic analysis by language experts.

Dysarthrias (impairments in the physical articulation of speech) are not included here.

- *Agrammatism*: loss of grammar (e.g. conjunctions such as **and**, **but**, **or** etc. along with contextual cues such as tense). Sometimes referred to as **telegraphic speech** (a contemporary analogue might be the 'texting speech' used with mobile phones). Individual words or phrases may be understood but not the overall meaning of what is being said. Present in certain dysphasias.
- *Akataphasia*: used by Kraeplin to describe (thought) disordered speech.
- *Alogia*: a functional (i.e. non-organic) inability to speak.
- *Asyndesis*[†]: a loosening of thought association.
- *Autism*: used by Bleuler to describe the fantasy-directed thought he believed to be characteristic of schizophrenia and schizoid personality. Normal thought is considered to be more reality-directed.
- *Bradylalia*: slowed speech.
- *Circumstantiality*: the conversation meanders via unnecessary details towards the eventual goal, describing all the circumstances up to and around the event in question whether or not they are relevant.
- *Clang association*: words are linked by sound (typically rhyming) or puns rather than syntax or meaning. An example of **loosening of association**.
- *Concrete thinking*: an inability to extrapolate beyond literal thinking or interpretation (as is required with abstraction, e.g. metaphors and proverbs).

- *Condensation*: two or more ideas are condensed into a new, incomprehensible idea.
- *Confabulation*: memories are unwittingly displaced in time and/or jumbled up with thoughts (e.g. something the subject only saw or heard, perhaps on television, is 'recalled' as a personal experience), often 'plugging gaps' caused by an organic amnesia (typically dementia).
- *Coprolalia*: the forced use of expletives (i.e. against the subject's will).
- *Derailment (Entgleisen)*[†]: theme of thought is regularly lost and replaced by something else.
- *Desultory*[*]: stream of thought in which ideas, correctly expressed in terms of syntax and grammar, are out of context and juxtaposed inappropriately.
- *Disorders of thought possession*: see **thought broadcast/insertion/withdrawal**.
- *Drivelling*[*]: components of thought are mixed up (faseln), losing all organization (**word salad**).
- *Dysphasia*: an impairment of language processing. Often sub-classified as either receptive (understanding language) or expressive (generating language).
- *Dysphonia*: impaired ability to vocalize.
- *Echolalia*: subject automatically repeats what someone else has just said.
- *Echologia*: repetition of another's speech using one's own words or phrases (i.e. not exact as in echolalia).
- *Flight of ideas*: pathologically high rate of change of thought. A degree of **loosening of association** and **pressure of speech** is usually implied.
- *Formal thought disorder*: the form (or structuring) of thought is impaired. The term (an abbreviation of schizophrenic formal thought disorder) is usually restricted to the more severe end of the resulting spectrum of abnormality, which ranges from **circumstantiality** through **loosening of association** to eventual **word salad**. Sometimes divided into 'positive' FTD (a failure to inhibit e.g. flight of ideas) and 'negative' FTD (a failure to express e.g. alogia).
- *Fusion (Verschmelzung)*[*]: interweaving (fusion) of two differing streams or elements of thought.
- *Interpenetration*[†]: separate themes of thought permeate each other, becoming reciprocally pervasive.
- *Knight's move*: a reference to the chess-piece that can change direction while moving. The term is used to describe an unexpected and drastic change in the direction of conversation ('knight's move thinking/speech'). Similar to **derailment**.
- *Logoclonia*: repetition of the last word's last syllable. Form of **perseveration**.
- *Logorrhoea*: voluble, garrulous, fluent speech (**pressure of speech**).
- *Loosening of association*: Bleuler considered this to be the central feature of schizophrenic thought disorder. It describes impaired cohesion or 'connectedness' between contiguous thoughts along clear semantic lines. Part of the spectrum of **formal thought disorder**.
- *Magical thinking*: the mental linking of unrelated thoughts/events, e.g. crossing fingers when playing the lottery, making a wish etc. A feature of certain obsessional symptoms such as orderliness or counting.
- *Malapropism*: the substitution of a word by one which sounds similar but is different in meaning, often resulting in a ludicrous phrase or sentence.
- *Metonym*[†]: imprecise expression (i.e. an approximation) that resembles intended word or phrase.

- *Mutism*: loss of speech in clear consciousness. Elective (i.e. non-organic) mutism is sometimes seen in children.
- *Neologism*: a new 'made-up' word, or novel use of a familiar word.
- *Omission**: senseless omission of a segment of thought.
- *Overinclusion†*: an inability to adequately circumscribe a topic of conversation or retain meaningful boundaries. Often used interchangeably with circumstantiality.
- *Palilalia*: rapid automatic repetition of a word or phrase over and again; a form of verbal **perseveration**.
- *Paralogia*: the verbal manifestation of (positive) formal thought disorder (i.e. thought disordered speech).
- *Paragrammatism*: term that overlaps with **agrammatism** and **paraphasia**.
- *Paraphasia*: incorrect substitution of a word with one that is related to it, usually in meaning (semantic paraphasia) or sound (phonetic paraphasia or malapropism). The incorrect word may or may not exist.
- *Perseveration*: organic disorder (typically frontal lobe dysfunction) characterized by the repetition of a response beyond its initial relevance, probably through a failure to suppress it appropriately.
- *Poverty of speech/thought*: decreased rate and quantity of thought. Speech is interspersed with long gaps, particularly when formulating a response.
- *Pressure of speech/thought*: increased rate and quantity of thought. Speech is rapid and difficult to interrupt. A degree of **loosening of association** is usually implied.
- *Prolixity*: in psychiatry, embellished verbosity verging on **flight of ideas**.
- *Psychomotor retardation*: slowed mental processing, resulting in slowed speech and action.
- *Schizophasia (word salad, speech confusion)*: words are jumbled up such that overall speech is difficult or impossible to understand.
- *Spoonerism*: swapping the initial letter(s) of two words in a phrase or sentence.
- *Stammer*: involuntary pauses, repetition or prolongation of word sounds, interrupting the flow of speech. May be accompanied by grimacing (in effort to 'get words out') and is more marked when anxious. **Stuttering** is a type of stammering characterized by the intermittent repetition of syllables during the course of speaking.
- *Stereotypy*: subject makes frequent use of a particular (but unnecessary) word or phrase in their general speech. May be normal as part of a colloquialism or dialect.
- *Stock word*: one that is regularly used in a different manner to its usual significance or meaning (as a component of **stereotypy**), e.g. 'right' or 'man'.
- *Substitution**: main thought or idea is replaced by a subsidiary one.
- *Tangentiality*: pursuing an incidental topic beyond its relevance to the overall theme of conversation ('going off on a tangent').
- *Thought block (entgleiten)*: thought is inexplicably and suddenly 'shut off' and may be described as the mind going blank. Objectively similar to thought withdrawal (sudden stop mid-speech); need explanation by subject to distinguish the two phenomena.
- *Thought broadcast*: the experience of failing to physically contain one's thoughts such that others can be aware of and participate in them (not 'mind-reading'). In some texts the failure of containment is described as a passive 'leak' and in others as an active 'broadcasting'.
- *Thought insertion*: the intrusion of thoughts into one's experience from an external agency.

- *Thought withdrawal*: the removal of one's thoughts by an external agency.
- *Verbigeration*: extreme formal thought disorder in which words and phrases become fragmented and unintelligible.
- *Vocal tic*: the paroxysmal outburst of non-purposeful sounds, words or phrases despite attempts to suppress them.
- *Vorbeireden (vorbeigehen)*: used by Ganser to describe talking 'past the point'; subject gives incorrect answers that nevertheless seem to suggest the question has been understood.

* part of classification of thought disorder proposed by Schneider.
[†] part of classification of thought disorder proposed by Cameron.

PHENOMENOLOGY OF EMOTION

Affect is the immediate, apparent emotional state. Mood is aligned with personality and is the more enduring, pervasive emotional state. 'Observed' or 'objective' mood is sometimes used interchangeably with affect.

- *Abulia*: loss of volition/decisiveness.
- *Alexithymia*: impaired ability to describe one's emotions.
- *Anhedonia*: impaired ability to enjoy activities that would normally be pleasurable.
- *Anosodiaphoria*: emotional indifference to disease.
- *Anxiety*: an unpleasant feeling of anticipatory tension.
- *Apathy*: loss of motivation.
- *Asthenic*: the common interpretation of this term is 'inadequacy' (weak-willed, hypochondriacal, prone to complaining) as one of Schneider's 10 psychopathic personalities. However, it was also used by Kretschmer (see Chapter 4) and in addition is associated with several entries in the ICD-10 (F06.6, F45.30, F60.7).
- *Belle indifference*: dissociation of affect in which the subject appears indifferent to their malady.
- *Blunting/flattening of affect*: degree of emotional expression is diminished. Sometimes used interchangeably with restricted affect.
- *Cyclothymia*: subject's mood cycles 'up and down' over a period of time. Swings are not as extreme as those of bipolar disorder.
- *Delusional mood/atmosphere/intuition* (also **apophanous mood** or **Wahneinfall**): a pervasive and compelling sense of being on the verge of some personally significant (and usually sinister) knowledge or event, often relieved by the onset of a delusion.
- *Dysphoria*: unpleasant mood.
- *Elation/euphoria*: abnormally high affect or mood.
- *Euthymia*: neutral mood (i.e. no deviation of mood such as elation, depression, anxiety etc.). Often used to denote 'normal' mood.
- *Guarded*: subject feels interrogated on interview and is reluctant to give information. A degree of **paranoia** is usually implied.
- *Incongruity of affect/mood*: inappropriate dissonance between an individual's mood and their circumstances or topic of conversation.
- *Lability of mood*: mood tends to fluctuate with unusual rapidity. Extreme lability of mood with total loss of emotional control is termed **emotional incontinence**.

- *Moria/Witzelsucht*: fatuous affect; apathy and silliness combined with general indifference (typically as a result of frontal lobe dysfunction).
- *Perplexity*: a psychotic subject appears to have the vague and troubling experience that something may be wrong with them. Possibly indicates a degree of **insight** on the periphery of their awareness too subtle for them to grasp.
- *Restricted affect*: the number of emotional responses is diminished. Often used interchangeably with blunting of affect.
- *Verstimmung*: ill-humoured mood state ('moodiness'). Associated depressive symptoms may 'rub off' on others, making them unhappy as well.

PHENOMENOLOGY OF AWARENESS

All dissociative (not aware of something that is there) and certain psychotic (aware of something that is not there) states could, at least in part, be considered disorders of awareness.

- *Automatism*: action without intent (i.e. an involuntary movement while seemingly conscious). May be simple or complex, inappropriate or out of character. The subject lacks (or partially lacks) awareness of, and subsequent recollection for, the event.
- *Clouding of consciousness*: organic state characterized by an impaired ability to mobilize, focus and sustain one's attention, resulting in disorientation and a reduced ability to respond and interact appropriately. Arbitrarily regarded to be a less severe state than delirium.
- *Coma*: a state of unconsciousness secondary to an organic cause (typically with a Glasgow Coma Scale ≤8).
- *Delerium*: toxic (i.e. secondary to an organic insult) confusional state characterized by fluctuating consciousness, disorientation and poor executive functioning (dementia is a global impairment of executive functioning in clear consciousness). Subjects are usually restless and bizarre in manner.
- *Depersonalization*: subject experiences being somehow detached from themselves such that their thoughts, sensations, body awareness, time perception etc. seem in some way unreal. Subject does however 'own' the low mood and/or anxiety that invariably accompanies this phenomenon, motivating them to seek help.
- *Derealization*: subject experiences themselves as being somehow detached from reality, such that their environment (including other people) lacks a certain indefinable 'genuineness' or 'completeness'. Depersonalization and derealization are regarded to be disorders in the experience of reality rather than psychotic symptoms, though they may occur in psychotic states.
- *Insight*: objective understanding of one's own psychological/mental state. Typically used in mental health services to describe the degree of agreement between a professional and their patient.
- *Oneiroid (dream-like) state*: subject experiences, and to some extent participates in, a 'dream' despite appearing awake and maintaining some awareness of their surroundings. Frequent and marked changes in affect and behaviour may occur as the subject experiences shifting perceptions and spatial or temporal orientations. Clinical presentation may be similar to delirium but the term is generally used in non-organic states or epilepsy.

- *Stupor*: markedly reduced physical and verbal reactivity to one's surroundings. Subject may appear to be fully alert or to have a reduced level of consciousness. Can occur in functional (e.g. dissociation) or organic (e.g. drug-induced) states.
- *Torpor*: subject is drowsy with reduced awareness and falls asleep readily.
- *Twilight state*: a prolonged oneiroid-like state but usually with organic causation (typically epilepsy). Characterized by a clearly defined start and finish, variable duration and unpredictable (possibly violent) behaviour.

PHENOMENOLOGY OF BELIEF

- *Ideas of reference*: subject believes events in the world (as relayed by newspapers/ TV etc.) are somehow aimed at, i.e. refer to, themselves. ↑Implausibility or fixity imply delusions of reference (sensitver Beziehungswahn).
- *Overvalued idea*: An excessively intense and pervasive preoccupation that, although regarded to be justified by the subject, is nevertheless partially or temporarily amenable to counter-argument or evidence (and so not of delusional fixity). The belief itself is not one that is usually held by others with a similar background.
- *Delusion*: An unshakeable ill-founded (i.e. unreasonable) belief, based on ill-founded reasoning given the subject's culture or background (note that over-valued ideas are preoccupying; delusions may not be). Although almost always false, delusions are distinguished by their abnormal reasoning and fixity rather than their lack of veracity; the subject's actual assertion may, by sheer coincidence, be correct. However, there is invariably a clear (and typically bizarre) discrepancy between the absolute conviction of the belief and the subject's actual (objective) evidence for it.

Types of delusions:

1 **Primary (autochthonous)**: arises without any apparent cause (i.e. without antecedent) and is therefore objectively incomprehensible. Sometimes follows a period of delusional mood. The subject does not experience him/herself as a single whole person (in mind and/or body) but as a composite of self and non-self
2 **Secondary**: understandable given the subject's prior mental state or circumstances (i.e. with antecedent), e.g. delusions of grandeur in context of manic state
3 **Delusional perception (apophanous perception)**: a correct perception is given (not necessarily straight away) a delusional and utterly incomprehensible (in terms of the subject's prior mental state) meaning. A type of primary delusion
4 **Delusions of control (passivity phenomena)**: aspect(s) of oneself (thoughts, images, emotions, volition) are attributed to an external agency (not merely influenced or controlled 'as if' by an external agency). During these so-called 'made' experiences subjects lose their sense of autonomy and believe they are no longer in charge of some aspect(s) of themselves
5 **Delusional misinterpretation**: subject attaches a delusional meaning to a correct percept in the context of a pre-existing delusion or other pathological mental state (a 'secondary delusional perception', though this expression is not used)
6 **Delusional memory**: the spontaneous 'recollection' of a false (and typically bizarre) experience which is believed by the subject to be true. If the recollected event actually occurred and was only later ascribed a delusional meaning, the subject is experiencing a delusional percept (if primary) or a delusional misinterpretation (if secondary).

- *Partial delusion*: Rarely used term describing a 'weakening' delusion as it gradually resolves. The recovered subject may or may not regain insight.
- *Paranoia*: subject believes the conversations/actions of others pertain to them, i.e. are personal. If the others are thought to intend distress/harm, the paranoia is persecutory in nature (if the persecution is attributed to an authority, resulting in frequent/aggressive complaints or lawsuits, this is termed a **querulent** delusion); alternatively it may be grandiose. ↑Implausibility or fixity imply delusional paranoia.

PHENOMENOLOGY OF PERCEPTION

Perceptual distortion: threshold and/or experience of a percept are altered due to abnormalities in sensory organs or pathways.

- *Hyper/hypoacusis:* changes in sensitivity to sound.
- *Macro (megalo)/micropsia:* visual changes with respect to size.
- *Dyschromatopsia:* colour distortion. Hallucinogens such as LSD can make colours seem especially vivid. Desaturation is suggestive of optic nerve disease.

Perceptual misinterpretation: an **illusion**; attributing a genuine sensation to an incorrect cause (e.g. misinterpreting a hanging coat to be an intruder). Contrast with delusional perception, in which a genuine sensation is first correctly perceived (i.e. sensed and interpreted) but then given some additional (delusional) significance. Types of illusion:

- *completion illusion*: incomplete/ambiguous percepts are interpreted incorrectly.
- *affect illusion*: emotional state effects interpretation of percept.
- *pareidolia*: vivid illusion heightened in intensity by focusing attention (e.g. seeing a face in the clouds). Affect and completion illusions are extinguished by attention.

False perception: a **hallucination**; subject experiences a perception in the absence of a stimulus but believes it to be genuine, i.e. they experience an imaginary stimulus as being real. A **pseudohallucination** is similar to a hallucination in all respects except that of absolute belief in the authenticity of the apparent stimulus (e.g. in terms of its spatial projection, 'solidity' vividness, etc.). An **eidetic image** is a perfect visual recollection ('photographic memory'). The subject does not regard an eidetic image to be the perception of a real stimulus (distinguishing it from a hallucination) and can suppress it by an effort of will (further distinguishing it from a pseudohallucination).

TYPES OF HALLUCINATION

- *Extracampine*: perception of something outside the normal sensory range (e.g. seeing things in another building or hearing voices from another city).
- *Functional*: a normal percept triggers an hallucination in the same modality. Both are experienced together and the hallucination is not merely a distortion of the percept (e.g. hearing angels' voices while listening to a water fountain).
- *Hypnogogic*: occurs whilst going to sleep. ⎫
- *Hypnopompic*: occurs whilst waking from sleep. ⎭ typically pseudohallucinations
- *Reflex*: a synaesthetic phenomenon. A normal percept in one sensory modality triggers an hallucination in another, e.g. 'seeing' music as it is heard.

HALLUCINATIONS IN SPECIFIC MODALITIES

AUDITORY

- *Elementary/simple*: basic sounds and noises. Tinnitus is a pseudohallucination since the subject does not believe it to be a genuine noise (similarly, so-called 'visions' are usually visual pseudohallucinations).
- *Complex*: voices (phonemes – Wernicke), music.
- *Voices*
  - *Own thoughts spoken aloud* (thought echo/sonorization): Gedankenlautwerden (thoughts and voices are synchronous) and echo de la pensé (voice is heard immediately after the thought). These terms often regarded as synonymous.
  - *Running commentary*: hallucinatory voice comments on person's actions.
  - First person ('I'), second person ('you' or address subject by name/directly; commands/imperatives; commentary), third person (refer to subject as 'he/she' or 'him/her'; usually involve more than one voice).
- *Palinacousis*: auditory perseveration. Subject may describe sounds and/or voices as 'echoing' for some time after the original stimulus has ended. A symptom of temporal lobe dysfunction, not psychosis.

PROPRIOCEPTIVE (BODY SCHEMA)

- *Vertigo* may be considered to be a vestibular hallucination movement.
- *Kinaesthetic*: hallucination of body or limb movement/position.
- *'Phantom limb'* (the continued awareness of a missing limb) is typically a proprioceptive pseudohallucination, and is often associated with pain. It is the opposite of hemisomatognosia, in which the subject experiences an intact limb as missing. In reduplicative phenomena subjects experience an additional limb or body part.

SOMATIC

- *Superficial*: involving sensations from skin, e.g. touch (haptic), temperature (thermic), liquid (hygric). Formication is the perception of insects crawling on, in or beneath the skin (characteristic of Ekbom's syndrome). Lhermitte's sign describes a sudden (typically <1 s) 'buzzing' or 'pins and needles' (paraesthesia) in the limbs and body on flexing the neck due to mechanical aggravation of damaged spinal nerves. Certain **dynias** are thought to be of predominantly psychological causation, such as unexplained itching, burning or pain of the skin, e.g. glossodynia (tongue), vulvodynia (vulva).
- *Deep*: visceral sensations, typically of a basic nature such as pushing/pulling/twisting. May be painful.

In coenestopathic states the subject experiences a qualitative change in the corporeality of a body part, i.e. a localized distortion of its material characteristics.

OLFACTORY AND GUSTATORY

May be prolonged and mood congruent. Suggestive of temporal lobe epilepsy though they can occur in functional psychoses. Dysgeusia is an impaired sense of taste.

VISUAL

- *Lilliputian*: hallucinations of miniature people and objects. Often associated with alcohol withdrawal and may be pleasurable.
- *Autoscopic*: visual hallucination of oneself. The subject may believe they have a double (Doppelganger). In negative autoscopy, subject cannot perceive their reflection in a mirror.
- *Experiential hallucinations*: visual hallucinations typically associated with temporal lobe epilepsy (thought to be vivid memories).
- *Phosphenes*: brief flashes of light usually perceived in a darkened environment or upon closing the eyes. May be induced by movement of the eyeball or a sudden noise. Indicative of a problem somewhere along the optic pathway.
- *Palinopsia*: visual perseveration (secondary to an organic cause).
- *Teichopsia* (fortification spectra): one of the temporary visual disturbances that sometimes precede a migraine, characterised by shimmering zigzag lines in the peripheral visual field.

ABNORMAL MOVEMENT/ACTION

Disorders of central causation are listed.

VOLUNTARY PURPOSEFUL MOVEMENT

- *Mannerism*: a 'normal' movement carried out unnecessarily frequently (e.g. blinking, flicking one's hair etc.). Manneristic postures are habitual poses that are exaggerations of the normal or adopted with excessive frequency.
- *Dyspraxia*: impaired ability to execute a familiar task despite intact coordination, sensation and motor pathways.
- *Compulsive act*: an unnecessary action executed as a release of rising inner tension to do so. The action is usually a particular task, whereas a motor tic is usually just a particular movement.
- *Pica*: persistent eating of any non-nutritive substance, e.g. geophagy (eating clay or soil). Associated with pregnancy, eating disorders (including anorexia and bulimia) and iron-deficiency anaemia. Formerly called cissa.

VOLUNTARY NON-PURPOSEFUL MOVEMENT

- *Stereotypy*: 'abnormal' (in as much that it serves no purpose) movement that is carried out with excessive frequency (e.g. foot-tapping, rocking), usually to the extent that it becomes characteristic for that person.
- *Tic*: a sudden, non-purposeful act that 'breaks through' despite attempts to suppress it. Can be simple (isolated movement of a muscle) or complex (coordinated movement of a group of muscles), and is usually characteristic for the individual. Worsened by stressful emotional states.

INVOLUNTARY PURPOSEFUL MOVEMENT

Hyper/hyporeflexia: e.g. exaggerated startle response in post-traumatic stress disorder (PTSD).

INVOLUNTARY NON-PURPOSEFUL MOVEMENT

- *Abasia*: difficulty walking. Astasia abasia is a dissociative disorder of gait.
- *Akathisia*: subject is compelled to keep moving due to an irresistible restlessness. In pseudoakathisia the subject appears to be akathisic but denies feeling restless.
- *Ambitendency*: subject is caught between executing and resisting an action.
- *Asterixis*: 'flapping' of the extended hands seen in liver encephalopathy.
- *Ataxia*: impaired coordination of gait.
- *Athetosis*: slow writhing movements of the trunk/limbs.
- *Automatic obedience (command automatism)*: subject carries out another's instructions without apparent subjective appraisal, i.e. regardless of consequences.
- *Ballismus*: the limb is thrown violently away from the body; an extreme form of chorea. Hemiballismis involves both limbs on one side of the body.
- *Blepharospasm*: strong contraction of the orbicularis oculi muscle(s). Typically intermittent (triggered by strong emotion, particular eye movements or bright light), but can progress to more or less continuous contraction.
- *Bruxism*: continuous gnashing or grinding of the teeth.
- *Catalepsy*: muscles are 'seized rigid' due to aberrant brain activity.
- *Cataplexy*: an abrupt loss of muscle tone as a result of sudden emotional change (as seen in narcolepsy), usually resulting in collapse.
- *Catatonia*: a psychotic symptom characterized by fixed/fluctuating extremes of activity (catatonic excitement) or inactivity (catatonic stupor).
- *Chorea*: irregular jerky movements of the trunk/limbs.
- *Cog-wheeling*: a term associated with the characteristic Parkinsonian sign of lead-pipe rigidity with superimposed tremor.
- *Copropraxia*: involuntary obscene gesticulation.
- *Dyskinesia*: 'abnormal movement' of organic origin. In psychiatry the term has become associated with neuroleptic-induced movement disorders (and so includes akathisias, dystonias, Parkinsonism, choreoathetosis etc.). The motor contingent of cranial nerves is characteristically affected – face (blepharospasm, orofacial/oromandibular, lip smacking), eyes (oculogyric crisis – a dystonic reaction of the extrinsic muscles), tongue (lingual dystonia with possible dysarthria or dysphagia), vocal cords (dysphonias), neck (torticollis or titubation) – but the peripheral nervous system is also commonly involved.
- *Dystonia*: recurrent prolonged (typically a minute or so) muscle contraction, causing abnormal movements or postures. Usually focal but can 'spread' to other parts of the body. The arched posture of opisthotonous is caused by spasm of the paraspinal musculature.
- *Echopraxia*: automatic mimicry.
- *Essential tremor*: familial or sporadic. Predominates in upper limbs but may progress to legs, head and neck. 4–8 Hz.
- *Forced grasping*: individual repeatedly grasps and shakes the offered hand despite instructions to the contrary.
- *Grimacing*: repeated baring of the teeth with erratic facial expressions.
- *Intention tremor*: worsens with purposeful movement (i.e. action with intention). Causes include cerebellar disease.
- *Lead-pipe rigidity*: a term associated with the hypertonicity of Parkinsonism.

- *Mitmachen*: form of automatic obedience in which the individual, despite being requested to resist, allows their body to be freely positioned. Upon release the body returns to resting position.
- *Mitgehen*: more extreme form of mitmachen, in which even the slightest pressure initiates movement.
- *Myoclonus*: sudden contraction of a muscle or muscle group. Can occur in isolation or as part of a generalized tonic–**clonic** seizure.
- *Negativism*: motiveless resistance to movement.
- *Nystagmus*: oscillation of the eyeball(s) around a particular axis (usually vertical, resulting in a swinging lateral gaze which does not necessarily cross the midline).
- *Obstruction (blocking)*: central disorder resulting in irregular hindrance of motor activity. Subject often reacts at the last moment.
- *Oculo-gyric crisis*: a dystonic upward (with or without lateral) gaze of the eyes.
- *Omega sign (crow's foot)*: characteristic furrowing of the brow (frowning) in depression.
- *Opposition (gegenhalten)*: attempts to move the subject result in an equal and opposite reaction, resulting in no net movement. Similar to negativism.
- *Parkinsonism*: the triad of bradykinesia (slowed initiation/execution/adaptation of movement), resting tremor and rigidity.
- *Perseveration*: persistence or repetition of a movement/verbal response beyond its relevance.
- *Physiological tremor*: normal, but can be exaggerated by emotional states, drugs (e.g. lithium/antidepressants), hyperthyroidism and alcohol withdrawal. Predominantly upper limbs, 8–13 Hz.
- *Posturing*: subject adopts bizarre or inappropriate postures for prolonged periods.
- *Psychological pillow*: subject holds their head a few inches above the floor/bed while lying on their back.
- *Resting tremor*: present at rest when limb is relaxed and supported.
- *Schnauzkrampf (snout spasm)*: the rounded lips are thrust forward in a tubular manner. Sometimes seen in catatonic schizophrenia and Klüver–Bucy syndrome.
- *Tardive dyskinesias*: a class of dyskinesias that tend to manifest late in neuroleptic therapy. Often disabling and may be irreversible. The actual movements are not necessarily any different from the more acute reactions.
- *Titubation*: tremor of the head (i.e. neck muscles).
- *Torticollis*: spasm of the sternocleidomastoid muscle resulting in a twisting of the neck.
- *Trismus*: spasm of masticatory muscles (lock-jaw).
- *Waxy flexibility*: subject's body has a plastic tone and can be moved into any position, which may then be held for a long time (flexibilitas cerea).

NAMED SYNDROMES

A syndrome is a characteristic pattern of signs and/or symptoms.

- *Capgras (illusion des sosies)*: delusional misidentification of familiar people as being impostors, i.e. exact doubles of the original. Can involve objects, e.g. furniture. More common in women, and usually associated with schizophrenia (except in elderly, in whom it tends to occur in isolation). Commoner than Fregoli syndrome.

In *intermetamorphosis*, subject has the delusion that people can physically change into each other.

- *Charles Bonnet*: vivid episodic visual hallucinations (typically involving animals/people in scenes), usually occurring in the elderly in clear consciousness with preserved insight and intellect. Possibly organic (often associated with visual impairments).
- *Cotard*: delusions of extreme hypochondriasis/loss/nothingness (nihilism), e.g. total poverty, rotting internal organs, being dead. May occur in psychotic depression; more common in elderly.
- *Couvade*: non-specific symptoms in a man that mimic those of his pregnant partner, most commonly in her 3rd and 9th months (he does not believe himself to be pregnant).

  Pseudocyesis is the presence of pregnancy symptoms (and sometimes certain signs, e.g. amenorrhea, abdominal distension, breast enlargement) in a non-pregnant woman who believes she is pregnant.
- *Da Costa*: somatization disorder focussing on the cardiovascular system.
- *de Cleramboult*: belief that another person (usually of 'higher' status and therefore inaccessible) is in love with the subject. Also termed erotomania. Note that wanting a sexual relationship with the other person is not necessarily a feature of this illness.
- *Dhat*: the attribution of a non-specific malaise to the passing of semen in the urine, believed to have been caused by excessive sexual activity.
- *Diogenes (senile self-neglect)*: describes the elderly subject who, in the absence of any apparent mental disorder, lives in extreme squalor.
- *Ekbom*: a hypochondriacal disorder of bodily infestation (typically of parasites crawling beneath/in/on the skin). May take the form of a delusion, tactile hallucination or over-valued idea.

  Rarely Ekbon's syndrome can also refer to a 'restless legs syndrome', a disorder in which the subject fidgets in order to alleviate odd sensations and discomfort in their legs. It is not synonymous with akathisia, which is a neuroleptic induced restlessness.
- *Fregoli*: delusional misidentification of strangers as familiar people; opposite of Capgras.
- *Ganser*: a dissociative state characterized by 'approximate answers'. Ganser originally also described hallucinations and altered consciousness as part of an organic disorder, but this full syndrome is very rare/disputed. More commonly, a partial 'Ganser state' may be seen as part of another disorder, such as schizophrenia.
- *Gerstmann*: organic disorder (dominant parietal lobe dysfunction) characterized by finger agnosia, right–left disorientation, dysgraphia and dyscalculia.
- *Gilles de la Tourette's*: combined vocal and multiple motor tic disorder.
- *Klüver–Bucy*: organic disorder characterized by visual agnosia, placidity (loss of aggression/fear), hyper-orality and hyper-sexuality.
- *Koro*: delusional disorder in chinese culture characterised by the belief that 'inappropriate' sexual activity has caused a potentially fatal imbalance in the subject's physical energies along with a shrinking of the penis back into the abdomen. Not to be confused with kuru which is a prior disease of the CNS.
- *Munchausen*: personality disorder characterized by the intentional production or feigning of symptoms. If symptoms are induced/complained of in a dependant (e.g. child), this is termed Munchausen by proxy.
- *Othello (morbid jealousy)*: delusions of partner's infidelity.

Neuroanatomy

9

CELLULAR COMPONENTS OF THE NERVOUS SYSTEM

The human nervous system consists of specialized cells called **neurones** (the functional units) and supporting cells called **neuroglia**.

Neurones: respond to stimuli with an electrical impulse that can be conducted over long distances.

Neurones have a cell body (**soma** or **perikaryon**) from which extend long processes in varying number. The latter can be an **axon**, of which there is usually one or many **dendrites**.

Axon (neurite; nerve fibre): stems from soma as **axon hillock** to become **initial segment**. These parts of the axon are devoid of intracellular inclusions such as Nissl granules (ribosomes) and it is from here that the **axolemma** commences. Axons vary in length and can be myelinated or not. Terminal enlargements form synaptic boutons. A single neurone may form up to 10 000 synaptic connections with as many as 1000 neurones. Sympathetic and parasympathetic axons terminate in thousands of **synaptic varicosities**. Axons convey information away from the cell body.

Dendrite: receives information from other cells through thousands of receptor contacts and has spines (12 μm diameter) that increase the cell surface area and are the sites of synaptic connection. Dendrites convey information towards the cell body.

Axons and dendrites contain similar cytoskeletal components (microtubules, actin filaments and neurofilaments); however, they differ significantly.

Nucleus: neuronal nuclei are spherical, central and 4–18 μm in diameter. Almost all neuronal nuclei have a **nucleolus** which is one-third their size and is necessary for protein synthesis.

Classification: neurones can be described as **unipolar (pseudo-unipolar)** (dorsal root ganglion cells of peripheral nervous system and those in trigeminal mesencephalic nucleus), **bipolar** (some olfactory and retinal cells and those in acoustic ganglion (VIII)), or **multipolar** (spinal motor neurones, cerebellar Purkinje cells, cortical pyramidal cells, neurones of autonomic nervous system) depending upon the number of axons and dendrites they possess. Most central nervous system (CNS) neurones are multipolar.

Alternatively, they can be described as amacrine (no axon), **Golgi type I** (long) or **Golgi type II** (short. 0.5–5 mm) according to axonal length.

Table 9.1 Comparison of axons and dendrites

Features	Axons	Dendrites
Morphology	Consistent diameter	Tapered
Arborization	Rare	Common
Conduction in relation to cell	Away	Towards
Numbers	Usually only one	Very many
Ribosomes	Nil	Yes
Cytoskeletal components	Neurofilaments > microtubules	Microtubules > neurofilaments
Specific proteins	Tau	MAP2

Golgi type I neurones form commissures, tracts and association/projection fibres. Golgi type II neurones remain within grey matter.

Neurones can also be described as afferent, efferent or interneurones.

- *Afferent neurones*: (sensory) mostly outside of CNS. Carry information towards spinal cord and brain.
- *Efferent neurones*: mostly outside of CNS. Autonomic efferents and motor neurones. Carry information to effector organs.
- *Interneurones*: originate and terminate within CNS. Ninety-nine per cent of neurones are interneurones.

NEUROGLIA (glial cells/glia)

First described by Virchow as nerve glue (neuro-glia). Glia make up 50 per cent of brain volume and outnumber neurones 10:1. Unlike neurones, glia are non-conducting and continually undergo mitosis. They are separated from neurones by intercellular spaces and fulfil a variety of functions.

Types:

ASTROCYTES

- maintain chemical environment and take up excess K^+
- structural support of nervous tissue
- part of blood–brain barrier
- involved in phagocytosis and healing
  - *protoplasmic astrocytes*: found mainly in grey matter, they have plenty of granular cytoplasm with a large nucleus and thick processes that flatten to form pedicles which adhere to neurones, blood vessels and pia mater.
  - *fibrous astrocytes*: predominantly in white matter, with longer but less branched extensions. Contain specific glial acidic fibrillary protein.

OLIGODENDROCYTES

- fewer branches and are smaller than astrocytes
- stained by del Rio–Hortega's silver method

- have numerous ribosomes and mitochondria and an extensive rough endoplasmic reticulum and Golgi apparatus
- synthesize myelin sheath (same as Schwann cells in peripheral nervous system)
- types:
  - interfascicular: white matter
  - perineuronal: grey matter
  - perivascular: white and grey matter.

MICROGLIA

Derived from haematopoetic stem cells; small with elongated nuclei and a paucity of cytoplasm. Found more in grey matter and from 10 per cent of total glia. Proliferate following injury, inflammation or degeneration and hence likened to macrophages (both express receptors for Fc portion of immunoglobulins).

EPENDYMA

Ciliated cells that line CNS cavities and aid cerebrospinal fluid (CSF) flow.
  Types:

- ependymocytes (ventricles and spinal cord central canal)
- choroidal epithelial cells (cover choroidal plexi)
- tanycytes (floor of third ventricle overlying median eminence).

NB special kinds of glia in:

- retina: **Muller cells**
- posterior pituitary: **pituicytes**
- cerebellum: **Bergman cells**.

NERVOUS SYSTEM DEVELOPMENT

Table 9.2 Embryonic derivation of central nervous system structures

Embryonic structure	Adult derivative	Ventricular component
Telencephalon (forebrain)	Cerebral hemispheres (cortex) Hippocampus Basal ganglia Olfactory bulb	Lateral ventricles
Diencephalon	Hypothalamus Thalamus Subthalamus Epithalamus	III ventricle
***Mes*encephalon**	Midbrain	Cerebral aqueduct (of Sylvius)
***Met*encephalon**	Cerebellum and pons	IV ventricle
***Mye*lencephalon**	Medulla	IV ventricle
Spinal cord	Spinal cord	Central canal

Third week of development – central nervous system appears as **neural** or **medullary plate** (elongated thickened plate of ectoderm) occupying anterior portion of embryonic disk.

- Lateral edges fold to form **neural folds** and central neural groove.
- Neural folds fuse to form **neural tube** which separates from overlying ectoderm.
- Coinciding with this is mesodermal somite segmentation (muscles and axial skeleton).
- Neural tube closure commences at level of 4th somite and proceeds in both directions until anterior and posterior neuropores remain.
- **Anterior neuropore** closes day 25.
- Neural tube divides to form the brain and its components and the spinal cord.
- Cephalic portion of neural tube forms the three primary brain vesicles:
  - **Prosencephalon** (forebrain)
  - **Mesencephalon** (midbrain)
  - **Rhombencephalon** (hindbrain).

Differential rates of growth result in constrictions and flexions:

- cervical flexure (junction of hindbrain and spinal cord)
- cephalic flexure (midbrain)
- pontine flexure (separates metencephalon and myelencephalon). Flexion is opposite to cervical and cephalic flexion.

(NB Alphabetical order of *mes, met, my*)
Fifth week of development:

- prosencephalon → telencephalon and diencephalon
- rhombencephalon → metencephalon and myelencephalon.

During gestation cortical neurones commence life cycle in close proximity to cerebral ventricles. Radial glial cells guide developing cortical neurones as they migrate (neuronal migration). Individual neurones stop migration at specific points and reach maturity developing dendritic and axonal connections.

CEREBRAL CORTEX (PALLIUM)

Grey matter (lacks myelinated nerve fibres and blood vessels): variable thickness (1.5 mm calcarine fissure to 4.5 mm motor cortex), contains 15 billion neurones.
Telencephalon forms three layers:

- outer *marginal* layer: cerebral cortex
- intermediate *mantle*: cerebral white matter
- inner *matrix* layer: surrounds lateral ventricles.

CORTICAL CELL TYPES

1 **Pyramidal cells**: most common, triangular cell bodies with apex pointing towards cortical surface. Vary in size 10–100 μm and found in all cortical layers

except molecular layer. Giant cells (Betz) feature of precentral gyrus (motor area 4).

2 **Stellate** (granule) cells: star-shaped and common with cell bodies of 4–8 μm. Present in all layers and greatest in layer IV.

3 **Fusiform** cells: usually spindle-shaped lying perpendicular to cortical surface and limited to deepest cortical layer.

4 **Horizontal cells of Cajal**: axis is parallel to cortical surface and are exclusive to molecular layer.

5 **Cells of Martinotti**: axon ascends from small cell body. Present throughout cortex but rare in molecular layer.

CORTICAL LAYERS

Hippocampal formation (archipallium) and olfactory cortex (paleopallium) have three layers and are called allocortex. Neocortex (neopallium) forms 90 per cent of cerebral cortex and consists of six layers:

  I **Molecular layer**: (plexiform layer) is outermost.

 II **External granular layer**: granular cells are Nissl-stained rounded cell bodies of stellate cells.

III **External pyramidal layer**: predominantly pyramidal cells.

IV **Internal granular layer**: contains thalamic myelinated nerve fibres called external band of Baillarger.

 V **Internal pyramidal layer**: Betz cells in precentral motor cortex. Internal band of Baillarger.

VI **Fusiform layer**: traversed by all fibres entering or exiting cortex.

CORTICAL MAPS

1905	Iain Campbell	20 areas
1909	Korbinian Brodmann	52 areas (Brodmann's areas (BA) still used)
1919	Cecile and Oscar Vogts	200 + areas
1929	Constantinou von Economo	109 areas

Cortex forms two convoluted hemispheres. Elevations are called **gyri**; depressions are called sulci. Deep **sulci** are called **fissures**. Each cerebral hemisphere consists of six lobes:

TO FLIP

Temporal
Occipital
Frontal
Limbic
Insular (central)
Parietal lobes

TEMPORAL LOBE

Lateral aspect consists of three gyri (superior, middle, inferior) bounded by two sulci (superior, inferior). Superior aspect consists of transverse temporal gyri of Heschl (posterior part on left side forms Wernicke's area BA 22). Anterior aspect forms temporal pole and medial aspect consists of hippocampus, entorhinal cortex, amydala and parahippocampal gyrus. The uncus and adjoining parts of the para-hippocampal gyrus contain the olfactory receptive area which when damaged can lead to anomia. Irritative lesions can also cause uncinate fits (occasionally feature olfactory hallucinations as aura).

Table 9.3 Temporal lobe lesions

Temporal lobe region	Effects of lesion
Medial	Anterograde amnesia
	L-side: verbal; R-side: non-verbal
Superior	L-side: Wernicke's sensory (receptive, fluent) aphasia;
	R-side: amusia
Posterolateral	L-side: semantic amnesia; R-side: prosopagnosia
Irritative lesion	Forced thinking, *déja vu, jamais vu*

Additional manifestations of temporal lobe dysfunction:

* upper homonymous quantrantanopia
* non-dominant lobe: dysprosody
* bilateral: Korsakoff's amnesia, Klüver–Bucy syndrome.

OCCIPITAL LOBE

Prominent calcarine sulcus on medial aspect.
Lobe contains primary visual cortex (BA 17) and association areas (BA 18 and 19).
Lesions inferior to calcarine fissure can lead to contralateral **hemichromatopsia**.
Additionally an L-sided lesion may cause dyslexia without agraphia.
Bilateral lesions superior to calcarine fissure can cause **Balint's syndrome**:

* optic ataxia (abnormal visual guidance of movements of limbs)
* oculomotor apraxia (inability to scan visual environment systematically)
* simultanagnosia (individual is unable to appreciate more than a single aspect of a stimulus configuration at any point in time; loss of panoramic vision; focus on central part of visual field).

Additional signs and symptoms of occipital lobe dysfunction: hallucinations and agnosias (prosopagnosia; visual agnosia; colour agnosia).

FRONTAL LOBE (See also Chapter 3)

Separated from parietal lobe by central sulcus (fissure of Rolando).
   Consists largely of medial and lateral aspects.
   Medial aspect divided into superior and inferior regions:

* *superior region* contains: anterior cingulate cortex and supplementary motor area
* *inferior region* contains: orbital cortex and basal forebrain.

Lateral aspect contains dorsolateral prefrontal cortex (DLPFCx) and frontal operculum which on dominant side contains **Broca's area** (BA 44 and 45).

Table 9.4 Frontal lobe lesions

Frontal lobe region	Effects of lesion
Superior medial aspect	Akinetic mutism
Orbital cortex	Personality changes: distribution, poor insight and judgement
Basal forebrain	Amnesia and confabulation
Dorsolateral prefrontal cortex	Impairment of cognitive and intellectual functions
Broca's area	Non-fluent, motor, expressive asphasia
Frontal operculum (non-dominant side)	Dysprosody
Irritative lesions	Eye deviation, amnesia

LIMBIC LOBE

Described by Willis as 'cerebri anatome' and by Broca (1878) as 'limbus' (border, ring) surrounding rostral brainstem and interhemispheric commissures. Lies beneath neocortex.

The limbic system can be defined according to development, function and connectivity, hence some disagreement about constituents:

Limbic system:

- limbic cortex
- limbic nuclei
  - subcortical
  - associated.

Limbic cortex COSH

- *C*ingulate gyrus – overlying corpus callosum (CC) (BA 24,32); allocortex
- *O*lfactory (primary) cortex
  - septal cortex
  - anterior perforated substance
  - prepyriform cortex (part of uncus of parahippocampal gyrus)
- *S*eptal cortex (septal region below septal nuclei CC genu)
  - septum pellucidum
  - subcallosal gyrus
- *H*ippocampal formation.

Subcortical limbic nuclei
Septal nuclei (beneath septal cortex)

- nucleus accumbens septi
- medial and lateral septal nuclei
- amygdala.

ABC
- *A*mygdala
- *B*asolateral amygdaloid (association with temporal lobe cortex)
- *C*orticomedial amygdaloid.

Associated limbic nuclei MERIT

- **M**ammillary body hyopothalamic nuclei
- **E**pithalamic habenular nucleus
- **R**eticular formation of midbrain tegmentum
- **I**nterpeduncular nucleus
- **T**halamic anterior nucleus.

Limbic system interconnections and circuits:

> Amygdala — *stria terminalis* → septal region — *longitudinal striae* → dentate gyrus → hippocampus

> Amygdala ← *diagonal band* — septal region ← *fornix* — hippocampus

Limbic system receives inputs from all sensory systems.
Limbic system outputs are mainly from amygdala or hippocampus.
Papez circuit (main hippocampal output) links limbic system and neocortex via cingulate gyrus.

> Hippocampus — *fornix* → mammillary body — *MTT* →
> → anterior nucleus of thalamus — IC → cingulate gyrus

multi-neuronal pathway

Amygdala output
|
stria medullaris
↓
habenular nucleus — *fasciculus retroflexus of Meynert* →
→ interpeduncular nucleus → reticular formation

Limbic system efferents:

- neocortex (conscious motor and sensory functions)
- hypothalamus (endocrine and autonomic function)
- brainstem reticular formation (arousal).

Limbic system lesions/stimulation effects:
Bilateral ablation of temporal lobe oral components (hippocampal formation, amygdala and uncus); causes **Klüver–Bucy syndrome**.
VaPOrS

> **V**isual **a**gnosia
> **P**lacidity (loss of aggression/fear)
> Hyper-**Or**ality (oral tendencies)
> Hyper-**S**exuality (increased drive).

Limbic system lesions (especially mammillary body haemorrhage) cause failure of memory consolidation. Seen in Korsakoff's syndrome (poor anterograde memory).
Stimulation of:

- septal areas: diminishes aggression
- amygdala: promotes aggression and oral actions (biting, licking, swallowing).

Hippocampal formation
- hippocampus (Ammon's horn)
- dentate gyrus
- subicular complex (component of parahippocampal gyrus, PHG).

Hippocampus: three principal layers.

- **plexiform layer**: alveus (white matter) – contains pyramidal cell axons and afferent neurones and forms ventricular surface of hippocampal formation
- **pyramidal layer** – contains pyramidal cells
- **polymorphic layer** – pyramidal cell main hippocampal cell; basket cells lie in proximity to pyramidal cells.

Stratum radiatum, lacunosum and moleculare are secondary laminae and comprise the **molecular layer**.
Stratum oriens consists of basket cells and basal dendrites.
Alveus axons form fimbria which form crura of fornix.

- *Parahippocampal gyrus* (PHG) (BA 28, enthorinal cortex): demarcated by collateral sulcus and continuous anteriorly with uncus, its superior aspect forms the subiculum. PHG has six-layer structure (neocortex). Subiculum along with hippocampal formation and dentate gyrus has three-layer structure (allocortex).
- *Dentate gyrus*: extends from indusium griseum to uncus between PHG and fimbria.
- *Indusium griseum*: (supracallosal gyrus, longitudinal striae): vestige of hippocampal formation.

INSULAR (CENTRAL) LOBE (ISLAND OF REIL)

Lies deep in **lateral (sylvian) fissure** and is circumscribed by circular sulcus.
Consists of long (posterior) and short (anterior) **oblique gyri** and a small medial projection to the anterior perforated substance called the **limen insula**.
Involved in autonomic functions and taste.

Substantia nigra (SN)
Anatomically consists of two parts – pars compacta and pars reticulata. Pars compacta is darker (contains neuromelanin) and contains more neurones.
SN afferents from:

- striatum (the majority) (GABA)
- pallidum (GABA)
- nucleus coeruleus (NA)
- raphe nuclei (5-HT)
- subthalamic nucleus (glutamate).

SN efferents to:

- striatum
- thalamus
- superior colliculus
- reticular formation.

PARIETAL LOBE

The postcentral and intraparietal sulci divide the lobe into:

- *Postcentral gyrus (sensory cortex)* (BA 3,1,2): somatotopic somatosensory area responsible for somesthesis (touch), vibration sense, kinesthesis (position) and epicritic touch (two-point discrimination).
- Posterior to postcentral gyrus are the *superior and inferior parietal lobules* (BA 7, part of 5 and 40); somatosensory association area involved in processing, realizing and storing sensory experiences.
- *Supramarginal* (BA 40) *and angular gyrus* (BA 39); components of inferior parietal lobule involved in reception and organization of language (particularly dominant hemisphere).
  - bilateral: astereognosia
    agraphognosia
    autotopagnosia
  - unilateral: dominant parietal lobe – finger agnosia; alexia with agraphia ± apraxia right–left disorientation; pain asymbolia ideomotor apraxia
    non-dominant parietal lobe – sensory inattention (neglect) i.e. anosognosia dressing apraxia; constructional apraxia geographic disorientation.

Table 9.5 Parietal lobe lesions

Parietal lobe region	Effects of lesion
Post central gyrus	Sensory loss
Optic radiation	Lower homonymous quadrantanopia
Non-dominant	Apraxia, anosognosia
Dominant	Gerstmann's syndrome
Inatative lesion	Somatic hallucinations

'**Gerstmann's syndrome**' (dominant parietal lobe):

- agraphia
- right–left disorientation
- finger agnosia
- aculculia
- alexia.

BASAL GANGLIA (BG)

These subcortical telencephalic grey masses consist of neurones and intermingled axons. The internal capsule separates the BG from the diencephalon. The BG are:

1 **corpus striatum** = caudate nucleus and = putamen (shell) and lenticular (lentiform) globus pallidus (pale nucleus globe)
2 **amygdaloid nuclear complex** (amygdala)
3 **claustrum**.

NB striatum (neostriatum) = caudate nucleus plus putamen (i.e. corpus striatum minus globus pallidus)

paleostriatum = pallidum = globus pallidus

BG CONNECTIONS AND PATHWAYS

- afferents to neostriatum, cerebral cortex, thalamus
- afferents to globus pallidus, neostriatum, subthalamic nucleus
- efferents from neostriatum, globus pallidus and substantia nigra
- efferents from globus pallidus, subthalamus, thalamus, hypothalamus, reticular formation, substantia nigra.

SIGNS OF BASAL GANGLIA LESIONS

Origin of extrapyramidal tract which modulates motor activity and tone.

Extrapyramidal tract fibres act within central nervous system and on corticospinal tract and not on lower motor neurones or spinal cord.

Basal ganglia damage results in involuntary movement disorders:

- parkinsonism, chorea, athetosis, hemiballismus.

FRONTAL-SUBCORTICAL CIRCUITS

Parallel circuits connecting frontal cortex, BG and thalamus (see Table 9.6):

Table 9.6 Frontal-subcortical circuits

Circuit (modal)	Function
Motor	Motor
Oculomotor	Eye movements
Dorsolateral prefrontal	Cognition
Anterior cingulate	Motivation
Lateral orbitofrontal	Personality

Neurology

10

CRANIAL NERVES

I OLFACTORY NERVE

1° neurones: nasal mucosa olfactory receptors communicate via cribriform plate of ethmoid bone.

2° neurones: olfactory bulb mitral cell axons pass to trigone via olfactory tract and lateral olfactory striae to reach primary olfactory area.

3° neurones: connect to olfactory association area. Anterior PHG (BA 28).

Anosmia causes:

*   *common*:
    - head injury
    - olfactory groove meningioma
*   *rare*:
    - frontal lobe tumour
    - obstructive hydrocephalus.

II OPTIC NERVE (see Figure 10.1)

1   **Retinal lesions** can cause scotomata or tunnel vision:
    - glaucoma
    - papilloedema
    - retinitis pigmentosa
    - *SCOTOMA*
        Sensile macular degeneration
        Compression of nerve
        Optic neuritis
        Toxins (tobacco)
        Olfactory groove meningioma
        Malignancy (optic n. glioma)
        Alcohol (thiamine deficiency).
2   **Optic nerve lesions** – those of:
    - scotoma
    - papilloedema

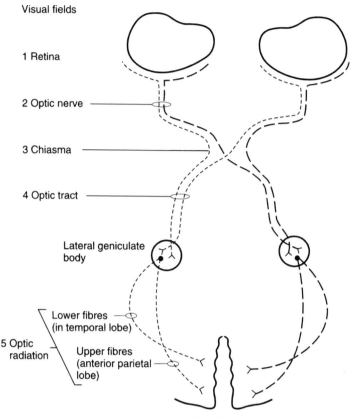

Figure 10.1 Visual pathways

  – ischaemia
  – syphilis.
3 **Chiasma lesions** cause:
    – unilateral/bilateral temporal hemianopia
    – *p*ituitary tumour (u*p*per fields affected first)
    – craniopharyngioma (lower fields affected first)
    – aneurysm.
4, 5 and 6 **Lesions of optic tract, radiation and cortex** cause homonymous hemi-
    anopias and quadrantic defects (usually ischaemia or tumours).
    Optic tract lesions often lead to incongruous visual fields.
    Optic radiation lesions do not show macular sparing.

When optic radiation lesions produce quadrantopias:

- *upper outer defect* is caused by lesion in the contralateral anterior temporal lobe
- *lower outer defect* is caused by a parietal lobe lesion.

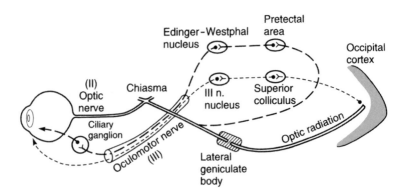

Accommodation reflex (--): involves the cortex
Light reflex (—— ——): does not involve lateral geniculate body or cortex
Convergence originates in cortex and is relayed to pupils via III n. nuclei
and oculomotor nerves.
Relaying of consensual reflexes takes place at brainstem level

Figure 10.2 Visual reflexes

*T*emporal – *T*op
Occipital cortex lesions show macular sparing because usually due to post cerebral
   artery infraction
*M*acular region supplied by *M*iddle cerebral artery

EYE REFLEXES (See Figure 10.2)

Light reflex:

> Retina — *optic n.* → pretectal area — (crossed) →
> → Edinger–Westphal nuclei — *III n.* → ciliary ganglion →
> → sphincter pupillae

Accommodation reflex:

> Retina — optic n. → Lateral geniculate body (LGB) —
> — optic radiation → cortex → superior colliculus →
> → III n. nucleus — III n. → eye muscles

NB Ac*co*mmodation reflex is *co*rtical. Light reflex is brainstem based.

PUPILS

III OCULOMOTOR NERVE

Two motor nuclei:

- somatic efferent nerve – supplies ocular muscles other than lateral rectus and superior oblique

Table 10.1 Pupil pathology

Pupil	Reaction to light	Causes
Small	Yes	Horner's syndrome, senile miosis
Small	No	Miotic drugs, opiates, Argyll Robertson, pontine haemorrhage
Large	Yes	Holmes–Adie, anxiety
Large	No	Mydriactic drugs, III n. palsy, midbrain haemorrhage, brain death

• Edinger–Westphal nucleus – parasympathetic supply to ciliary muscles and constrictor pupillae.

Lesions: paralysis of eyelid. Eye is deviated down and out. Pupil dilated with no response to light (physical cause). Normal pupil suggests parasympathetic fibres spared as in diabetes.

IV TROCHLEAR NERVE

Supplies superior oblique.
Lesions: failure of downward gaze during adduction.

V ABDUCENS NERVE

Supplies lateral rectus.
Lesion: Commonest ocular palsy. Eye deviated towards nose.
Causes of III, IV and VI nerve palsies: vascular, neoplasm, raised intracranial pressure, diabetes, multiple sclerosis, encephalitis.

VI TRIGEMINAL NERVE

Largest cranial nerve with four nuclei:

• mesencephalic nucleus (proprioception)
• main sensory nucleus (touch)
• spinal nucleus (pain and temperature)
• motor nucleus.

SENSORY COMPONENTS

Three sensory nuclei receive sensations via three main branches:

• ophthalmic nucleus: frontal, lacrimal and nasociliary nerve branches supply: upper eyelid, anterior scalp, lacrimal gland, lateral conjunctiva, eyeball, nasal skin and mucosa
• maxillary nucleus: infraorbital, superior alveolar and zygomatic nerve branches supply: upper teeth, cheek, roof of mouth and soft palate

- mandibular nucleus: auriculotemporal, buccal, inferior alveolar and lingual nerve branches supply: skin of temple and cheek, lower lip, teeth and chin and anterior two-thirds of tongue.

MOTOR COMPONENT

Supplies:

- muscles of mastication (massesters and pterygoids)
- temporalis.

  Reflexes:

- *Corneal reflex*: earliest to be affected. Afferent of corneal touch is unilateral trigeminal (ophthalmic), efferent (bilateral blink) is bilateral facial nerve.
- *Jaw reflex*: hyper-reflexia indicative of upper motor neurone lesion.
- *Glabbelar tap*: blinking *p*ersists in *P*arkinson's.

  Damage due to demyelination, injury, tumour, infection.

VII FACIAL NERVE

Principal nuclei that serve three main functions:

- *Sensory nucleus of tractus solitarius* Receives taste sensation from anterior two-thirds of the tongue, hard and soft palate and floor of the mouth. Carried in chorda tympani (branch of VII nerve that joins trigeminal lingual nerve).
- *Parasympathetic nucleus* Secretomotor function for lacrimal, sublingual and submandibular other glands (test lacrimation with Shirmer's test).
- *Motor nucleus* Motor supply to facial muscles. Test by asking for a smile, closure of eyes tightly and to look up.

  Facial weakness Upper half of face has bilateral (additional contralateral) innervation. Therefore upper motor neurone lesion leads only to weakness of lower portion of face. Lower motor neurone lesion affects whole face. Common idiopathic cause (Bell's palsy).
  Facial nerve passes through facial canal in temporal bone, stylomastoid foramen and parotid gland. Branches of facial nerve: temporal, zygomatic, buccal, mandibular, cervical.

VIII VESTIBULOCOCHLEAR NERVE

Cochlear nerve: responsible for hearing.
Vestibular nerve: responsible for maintenance of balance/equilibrium.

Tests for deafness – using tuning fork (512 Hz):

- *Weber test* Tuning fork stimulated and placed at vertex
  - if hearing is normal sound appears to emanate mid-line
  - *conduction deafness* – sound louder in affected ear
  - *nerve deafness* – sound louder in normal ear
- *Rinne test* Normally air conduction is better than bone. Tuning fork stimulated and placed initially base upon mastoid bone and then fork is held in line with

meatus. Air > bone is normal Rinne-positive. If not then Rinne–negative, i.e. conduction deafness

- *conductive deafness*: wax, infection (otitis media)
- *perceptive deafness*: old age (presbyacusis), trauma, tumour, infection (mumps, rubella).

Inner ear or brainstem pathology can cause **vertigo** (unsteadiness with subjective sensation of rotation).

IX GLOSSOPHARYNGEAL NERVE

Has three major nuclei – motor, parasympathetic and sensory.
Plays role in sensory arc of **gag reflex**.
Also conducts taste from posterior one-third of the tongue.

X VAGUS NERVE

Has three major nuclei – motor, parasympathetic and sensory.
Motor supply to larynx and pharynx. Motor component of **gag reflex**.
Test by asking patient to say 'Aah'; if damaged, uvula moves to intact side.
Parasympathetic component important in visceral functions of heart, lungs, gastrointestinal tract.

XI SPINAL ACCESSORY NERVE

Cranial root: supplies larynx, pharynx and soft palate.
Spinal root: supplies trapezius and sternocleidomastoid muscles.

XII HYPOGLOSSAL NERVE

Supplies muscles of the tongue.
If nerve is damaged, upon protrusion tongue deviates to affected side.
Bulbar and *p*seudobulbar palsy Concern cranial nerves IX, X and XII.
Both lead to dysarthria and dysphagia.
Clinical distinction of u**pp**er motor neurone (UMN) and lower motor neurone (LMN) damage made on basis of signs (Table 10.2):

Table 10.2 Bulbar and pseudobulbar palsy

	Lower motor neurone (LMN) – bulbar	Upper motor neurone (UMN) – pseudobulbar
Speech	Nasal	
Tongue	Flaccid; fasciculation	Spastic; small for mouth
Jaw jerk	Normal or absent	Brisk
Emotions	Normal	Labile
Cause	Infections, syringobulbia	Stroke, demyelination

SPINAL CORD

40–45 cm in length. About 1 cm diameter. Extends from medulla oblongata to conus below which spinal nerve roots form cauda equina. Cervical and lumbar enlargements because of extra fibres for limbs.

31 spinal nerves emerge symmetrically either side of spinal cord and leave vertebral canal via intervertebral foramina. Each spinal nerve is formed from dorsal and ventral roots which unite within the intervertebral foramina to form the spinal ganglia. The 31 pairs of spinal nerves are grouped as follows (8 cervical; 12 thoracic; 5 lumbar; 5 sacral; 1 coccygeal).

PERIPHERAL NEUROPATHY (see Figures 10.3–10.5)

- Hypertrophic (p*ALPA*ble) neuropathy:
  - *A*cromegaly
  - *L*eprosy
  - *P*eroneal muscular atrophy (Charcot–Marie–Tooth)
  - *A*myloidosis
- Motor neuropathy (predominantly):
  - Guillan–Barré syndrome
  - lead poisoning
  - peroneal muscular atrophy
  - porphyria (acute intermittent)
  - diphtheria
  - herpes zoster
- Sensory neuropathy (predominantly):
  - nutritional deficiency (B12, folate)
  - amyloid
  - diabetes
  - uraemia
  - paraneoplastic
- *PAIN*ful neuropathy:
  - *P*oisoning (thallium)
  - *AIDS*-related neuropathy
  - *N*utritional.

BLOOD SUPPLY OF THE BRAIN

The brain receives blood from the internal carotid (branch of common carotid) and vertebral (branch of subclavian) arteries. The R and L vertebral arteries join at the level of the pons, ventral to the brainstem, to form the basilar artery. Branches from the basilar artery along with those from the internal carotid arteries form the circle of

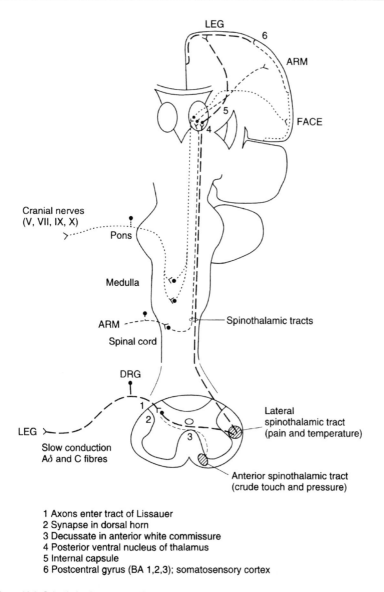

LEG

6

ARM

5

4

FACE

Cranial nerves
(V, VII, IX, X)

Pons

Medulla

ARM

Spinal cord

DRG

1

2

3

LEG

Slow conduction
Aδ and C fibres

Spinothalamic tracts

Lateral
spinothalamic tract
(pain and temperature)

Anterior spinothalamic tract
(crude touch and pressure)

1 Axons enter tract of Lissauer
2 Synapse in dorsal horn
3 Decussate in anterior white commissure
4 Posterior ventral nucleus of thalamus
5 Internal capsule
6 Postcentral gyrus (BA 1,2,3); somatosensory cortex

Figure 10.3 Spinothalamic sensory pathways

Willis at the base of the brain. The various branches and the parts of the brain they supply are shown in Figures 10.6 (p. 104) and 10.7 (p. 105).

If brain blood supply is compromised clinically it may lead to transient ischaemic attacks (TIAs) and cerebrovascular accidents (strokes). The signs and symptoms necessarily correspond to the parts of brain affected.

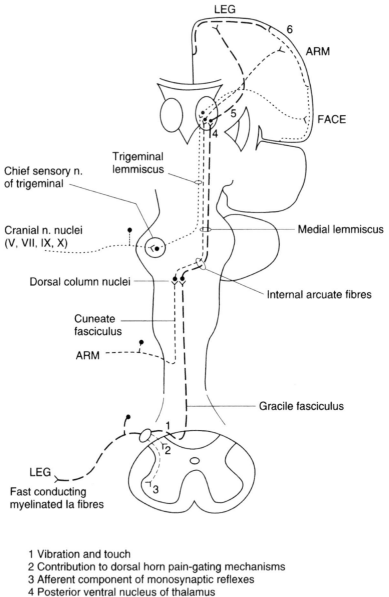

LEG

6

ARM

FACE

Trigeminal
lemmiscus

Chief sensory n.
of trigeminal

Medial lemmiscus

Cranial n. nuclei
(V, VII, IX, X)

Dorsal column nuclei

Internal arcuate fibres

Cuneate
fasciculus

ARM

Gracile fasciculus

LEG

Fast conducting
myelinated Ia fibres

1 Vibration and touch
2 Contribution to dorsal horn pain-gating mechanisms
3 Afferent component of monosynaptic reflexes
4 Posterior ventral nucleus of thalamus
5 Internal capsule
6 Somatosensory cortex

Figure 10.4 Dorsal column sensory pathways

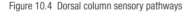

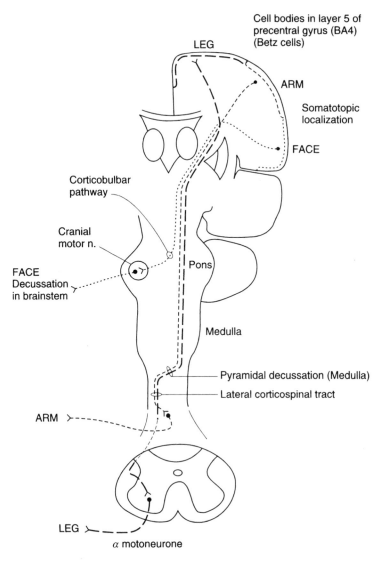

Figure 10.5 Spinal motor pathways

CAROTID ARTERY TIA SYMPTOMS AND SIGNS

- Amaurosis fugax (ipsilateral)
- Aphasia
- Contralateral hemiparesis
- Contralateral hemisensory loss
- Retinal artery emboli.

VERTEBROBASILAR ARTERY TIA SYMPTOMS AND SIGNS

- Dysarthria
- Dysphagia
- Vertigo
- Vomiting
- Circumoral paraesthesiae
- Drop attacks
- Tinnitus
- Transient global amnesia
- Nystagmus
- Ataxia.

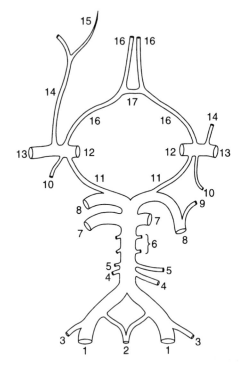

1 Vertebral	10 Anterior choroidal
2 Anterior spinal	11 Posterior communicating
3 Posterior inferior cerebellar	12 Internal carotid
4 Anterior inferior cerebellar	13 Middle cerebral
5 Labyrinthine (internal auditory)	14 Ophthalmic
6 Pontine	15 Central retinal
7 Superior cerebellar	16 Anterior cerebral
8 Posterior cerebral	17 Anterior communicating
9 Posterior choroidal	

Figure 10.6 Blood supply of the brain

ANTERIOR CEREBRAL ARTERIES

Supply:

- medial aspects of orbital, frontal and parietal cortex
- anterior part of internal capsule
- basal nuclei.

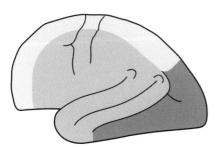

Surface pattern of
cerebral blood supply

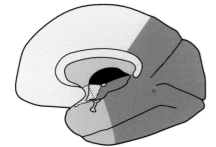

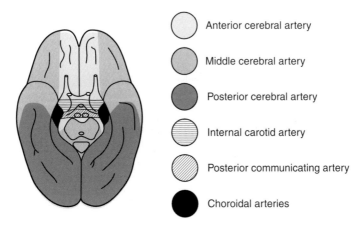

Figure 10.7 Surface pattern of cerebral blood supply

Interruption may lead to:

- contralateral lower limb motor weakness and sensory loss
- incontinence
- release of primitive reflexes (palmo-mental, snout, grasp)
- akinetic mutism (bilateral frontal lobe damage).

MIDDLE CEREBRAL ARTERIES

Supply:

- temporal, parietal and frontal cortex
- internal capsule
- basal nuclei.

Interruption may lead to:

- contralateral hemiplegia, hemianopia and sensory loss
- aphasia
- dressing apraxia
- contralateral neglect.

POSTERIOR CEREBRAL ARTERIES

Supply:

- inferior aspect of temporal and occipital (visual) cortex*
- posterior thalamus
- midbrain structures
- choroid plexus.

(*macular area of visual cortex supplied by middle cerebral artery.)
Interruption may lead to:

- *midbrain (Weber's) syndrome*
  - contralateral hemiplegia
  - III nerve palsy
- thalamic syndromes
- homonymous hemianopia with macular sparing
- anomia.

POSTERIOR INFERIOR CEREBELLAR ARTERY (PICA)

Occlusion leads to the **lateral medullary (Wallenberg's) syndrome**. It affects the brainstem and cerebellum and produces:

- Brainstem:
  - ipsilateral facial pain and temperature sensory loss*
  - laryngeal and pharyngeal (palatal) paresis because of damage to nucleus ambiguus
  - Horner's syndrome (ptosis and miosis) because of sympathetic fibre damage

  – contralateral limb and trunk pain and temperature sensory loss* (*together termed alternating hypalgesia).
- Cerebellum: *HAND*

  Hypotonia
  Ataxia (ipsilateral limb) due to cerebellar tract damage
  Nystagmus
  Dysarthria.

BASILAR ARTERY PARAMEDIAN BRANCH OCCLUSION (PENETRATING MIDLINE BRANCHES)

May result in a variety of syndromes:

- *pontine level*: Millard–Gubler syndrome
  – abducens (VI cranial nerve) and facial (VII cranial nerve)
  – palsy contralateral hemiplegia
- *midbrain level*: Benedikt's syndrome
  – oculomotor (III cranial nerve) palsy
  – contralateral tremor (red nucleus – cerebellar output)
- *medullary level*: 'locked-in' (de-efferentation) syndrome
  – (bilateral damage to anterior aspect of brainstem)
  – complete bulbar palsy – hence mute
  – interruption of corticospinal tracts leads to quadriplegia.

(NB retain ability to blink and move their eyes and are fully cognisant.)

VENTRICULAR SYSTEM

Consists of four communicating cavities within the brain. All are lined by ependyma and contain cerebrospinal fluid (CSF) produced from blood by the choroid plexuses within each ventricle.

There are two lateral ventricles (R and L) each communicating with a central third ventricle (III) via the interventricular foramen of Munro.

The third ventricle is connected to the ponto-medullary fourth ventricle (IV) via the cerebral aqueduct of Sylvius.

The fourth ventricle is continuous with the central canal of the spinal cord inferiorly and also communicates with the subarachnoid space via the **m**idline foramen of **M**agendie and the two **l**ateral foramina of **L**uschka (see Figure 10.8).

The choroid plexus is rich vascular tissue consisting of a network of pia mater blood vessels which project into each ventricle. Choroid plexus is covered by a layer of ependyma and secretes about 300–600 ml of CSF per day (NB ventricular volume is 25 mL and subarachnoid space volume is 110 mL). CSF is a colourless, clear, almost protein-free blood filtrate. It flows from the ventricles into the subarachnoid space and is eventually actively transported back into the blood circulation via superior sagittal sinus arachnoid granulations.

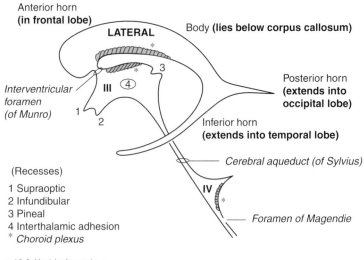

Figure 10.8 Ventricular system

CSF pushes the arachnoid layer against the dura creating the subarachnoid space between the pia mater and the arachnoid. Its principal function is to support and protect the brain against trauma.

HYDROCEPHALUS

1 **Non-obstructive**: communicating e.g. brain atrophy (Alzheimer's disease)
2 **Obstructive**: communicating e.g. Normal pressure hydrocephalus, meningitis, subarachnoid haemorrhage
3 **Obstructive**: non-communicating e.g. obstruction of CSF flow within ventricular system, cerebral aqueduct stenosis, tumour.

SIGNS OF CEREBELLAR LESIONS

Single hemisphere damage leads to ipsilateral signs and usually intact hemisphere compensates for and eventually assumes lost functions.

- Intention tremor (can be elicited with finger–nose or heel–shin test) with irregular rhythm (dysmetria)
- Dysdiadochokinesia
- Truncal ataxia
- Ataxic gait
- Dysarthria (scanning speech)
- Hypotonia.

DISORDERS OF GAIT

Cause	Gait
cerebellar	ataxia
normal pressure hydrocephalus	apraxia
Parkinson's disease	festinant gait
tabes dorsalis	steppage
stroke	hemiparetic gait (circumduction)

TESTS OF PSYCHOGENIC SIGNS AND SYMPTOMS

- *Psychogenic blindness*: eyes respond normally to spinning (vertically striped) cylindrical drum resulting in optokinetic nystagmus.
- *Psychogenic anosmia*: usually individual claims a complete loss of smell. However, normally despite damage to the olfactory nerve (e.g. following head injury) the detection of noxious stimuli, e.g. ammonia, is retained through trigeminal innervation.
- *Psychogenic weakness*: 'intermittent' as individual initially exerts some effort and then 'gives way'. Can be demonstrated with the face–hand test (patient prevents their falling hand from hitting their face) or by eliciting Hoover's sign (individual inadvertently pushes 'weak leg' downwards whilst raising unaffected leg and fails to press down normal leg when lifting 'weak' leg).
- *Psychogenic gait impairment*: astasia–abasia: individual staggers as if about to fall, grasping supports and people around them. In doing so they display balance, strength and coordination and do not usually fall.
- *Psychogenic sensory loss*: distribution of loss does not correspond to anatomical patterns of sensory innervation. Midline demarcation of loss is exaggerated.
- *Psychogenic amnesia*: individual claims of global loss of knowledge (including personal information), inability to acquire new information and scores less than predicted by chance on multi-choice recall.

MOVEMENT DISORDERS

PARKINSON'S DISEASE (PD) (JAMES PARKINSON 1755–1824)

Prevalence 1–2/1000 (1/200 age >70 years).

PARKINSONISM *IDiOPATHIc*

*I*diopathic (paralysis agitans) – commonest, insidious onset (age 50–60 years), with tremor often first sign. Progressive and initially asymmetrical presentation.

*D*rug *i*nduced – neuroleptics cause symmetrical slowness, rigidity and dystonic movements. Tremor less common.

Organic disorders – 'Parkinsonism plus': progressive supranuclear palsy; primary autonomic failure (Shy–Drager syndrome), olivopontocerebellar degeneration, Huntington's disease, Creutzfeldt–Jakob disease.

Post-encephalitic Parkinsonism – following encephalitis lethargica outbreaks (neurofibrillary changes are characteristic feature).

Atherosclerosis – occurs in setting of vascular disease (ischaemia, hypertension, stroke) presents mainly with rigidity and bradykinesia (little tremor). Poor response to medication.

Trauma – dementia pugilistica.

Hydrocephalus (normal pressure).

Intoxication – carbon monoxide, heavy metals, e.g. manganese, copper (Wilson's disease), MPTP (methyl phenyl tetrahydro pyridine – byproduct of illicit narcotic manufacture that specifically causes substantia nigra dopaminergic (DA) neurone degeneration).

PATHOLOGY OF IDIOPATHIC PD

NEUROPATHOLOGY

- Striatal loss of dopamine (putamen > caudate) (clinical presentation when DA loss >80 per cent).
- Melanin-containing cell bodies in pars compacta of substantia nigra undergo depigmentation (reduced pre-synaptic nigrostriatal DA production leads to diminished inhibition of striatal cholinergic neurones):
  - depigmentation of locus coeruleus and vagus dorsal motor nucleus.
  - ↓ cortical NA and that in locus coeruleus.
  - ↓ CCK and substance P in substantia nigra.
  - ↓ frontal cortex somatostatin.
  - Loss of neurones sometimes → diffuse cortical atrophy.
  - Reactive astrocytosis.
- Lewy bodies (amorphous, electron-dense bodies with proteinaceous core) – found in many structures but in particular: substantia nigra, locus coeruleus and dorsal motor nucleus of vagus.
  - Not characteristic of post-encephalitic PD or chemically induced parkinsonism.
  (NB occasionally found in normal brain tissue and Alzheimer's disease.)

CLINICALLY

Classic triad of tremor, rigidity and bradykinesia:

- 'Simian' stoop and festinant (shuffling) gait. Reduced arm swing.
- expressionless, unblinking, mask-like face maintaining 'serpentine' stare.
- greasy skin (seborrhoea), excessive salivation and slurred, soft, sonorous voice.
- small handwriting (micrographia).

PSYCHOLOGICAL COMPLICATIONS

- Depression (50 per cent) – guilt is less common a feature and suicide rate is low.
- Psychosis (10 per cent) – delusions and visual hallucinations.
- Dementia (15 per cent of all patients, 40 per cent of those >70 years old).
- Cognitive deficits – bradyphrenia, visuospatial impairments, poor memory (especially recent) and abstract reasoning.

HUNTINGTON'S DISEASE (HD) (GEORGE HUNTINGTON, 1850–1916)

1 in 20 000 males and females equally affected. Typical onset 25–50 years of age.

Autosomal dominant genetic disorder. Excessive trinucleotide CAG repeats on short arm of chromosome 4 (normally about 9–39 repeats; HD associated with >40 repeats; the greater the number of repeats the younger the onset of disease).

Results in abnormal protein called huntingtin.

It is thought that the genetic defect affects NMDA receptor function and that this predisposes to glutamate-induced excitotoxicity.

Neuropathology:

- cerebral cortex atrophy especially frontal lobes
- cortical neuronal loss affects layers III, V and VI
- neuronal degeneration and loss associated with marked astrocytosis
- ventricles are enlarged and are described as 'bat-wing ventricles'
- marked caudate nucleus atrophy, especially the head of the caudate. Begins medially and eventually interrupts cotico-striato-pallido-thalamic connections. Detectable by CT and MRI
- degeneration of striatal GABA neurones ($\downarrow$ caudate (GABA) to < 50 per cent of normal) and reduction of glutamic acid decarboxylase activity (striatal $\downarrow$ of up to 85 per cent)
- PET shows early (prior to structural changes) caudate hypometabolism
- loss of striatal encephalinergic neurones (project to globus pallidus) and substance P-containing neurones (project to substantia nigra)
- reduction in number of striatal aspartate receptors
- ACh levels $\downarrow$
- somatostatin and neuropeptide Y levels $\uparrow$
- DA hypersensitivity.

Clinically HD produces changes of *m*ood, *m*otion and *m*entation.

- *Initial symptoms*: 10 per cent in childhood and 25 per cent over the age of 50 years.
- *Emotional symptoms* include anxiety, depression and irritability. Occasionally paranoid psychotic symptoms.
- *Motor symptoms* include choreiform movements which are initially distal (piano-playing; milk-maid's sign; jack in the box tongue), abnormal saccades, dystonia, tremor, dysarthria abnormality of gait (lurching and contorted).
- *Cognitive symptoms* are those of insidious global dementia. Language function and memory are relatively spared.

WILSON'S DISEASE (HEPATOLENTICULAR DEGENERATION) (S. WILSON 1878–1936)

Autosomal recessive genetic disorder (chromosome 13).
 Caeruloplasmin (copper-carrying globulin) deficiency leads to copper deposition:

- *cerebrum*: dementia and emotional lability
- *putamen*: choreoathetosis, 'wing-beating' or 'bat-wing' tremor
- *liver*: cirrhosis, hepatosplenomegaly, jaundice
- *eye*:
  - cornea (Descemet's membrane)
  - lens (sunflower cataract)
  - cornea (Kayser–Fleischer ring – outer margin of iris).

Clinically *ABCDE*
*A*thetosis
*B*ehavioural changes
*C*ognitive impairment
*D*ysphagia, *D*ysarthria and *D*rooling
*E*motional lability.

TICS *PQRSt*

*P*urposeless, *Q*uick, *R*epetitive, *St*ereotyped movements of functionally related muscle groups.
 Described as simple (incomplete movements) or complex (complete movements) and can be motor or vocal. The frequency and intensity of tics is increased by anxiety, fatigue and excitement; however, they can be consciously temporarily suppressed. Occur three times more often in boys. Peak age of onset 7 years. Ninety per cent remit spontaneously within 5 years.

GILLES DE LA TOURETTE'S SYNDROME (ITARD 1825)

STUV
*S*tereotypes (jumping, dancing)
*T*ics
*U*tterances (clicks, throat clearing, snorts, grunts)
*V*ocal tics (coprolalia, occasionally accompanied by copropraxia).

Associated with:

- obsessive–compulsive symptoms (50 per cent)
- attention-deficit hyperactivity disorder (ADHD)
- soft neurological signs
- minor EEG abnormalities
- ↓ glucose metabolism (cingulate and inferior frontal cortex).

NEUROLEPTIC-INDUCED MOVEMENT DISORDERS

Acute onset: acute dystonia, oculogyric crisis, akathisia, Parkinsonism.

Tardive (late) onset: tardive dyskinesias, tics, oral-buccal-lingual syndrome, akathisia, dystonia, stereotypes.

Akathisia: regular, continuous leg movements (e.g. to and fro motion, crossing and uncrossing).

Tardive dyskinesia: irregular or stereotyped lower face, tongue and jaw movements. Associated with prolonged high-dose neuroleptic exposure and more common in women and with increasing age.

EPILEPSY (see Figure 10.9)

Lifetime prevalence 2 per cent.

Two-thirds partial (commonest temporal lobe epilepsy – TLE), remainder generalized and mixed.

CAUSES *ICTAL*

75 per cent *I*diopathic

9 per cent *C*erebrosvascular accident (CVA)

7 per cent *T*rauma

6 per cent *Al*cohol.

Other causes: drugs, infections, malformations, degenerative and metabolic diseases.

EPILEPTIC PERSONALITY *PERSON*

*P*edantic

*E*gocentric

*R*eligious

*S*low in thought ('viscous')

*O*bsessional

'k*N*it-picking' – critical.

PSYCHIATRIC ASPECTS OF EPILEPSY

- Ictal prodrome
  STIRS
  - ↓ *S*leep
  - ↑ *T*ension
  - ↑ *I*rritability
  - ↑ *R*estlessness
  - *S*uicidal ideation and depression

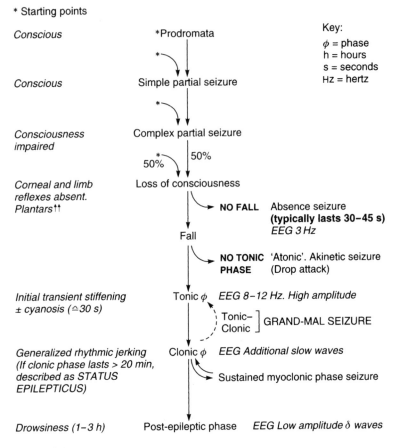

* Starting points

Key:
ϕ = phase
h = hours
s = seconds
Hz = hertz

Figure 10.9 Epilepsy

- Ictal: automatisms, fugues, twilight states
- Inter-ictal:
  - aggressive behaviour – **E**pisodic **D**yscontrol **S**yndrome:

    EEG changes, **D**isorder of personality, **S**enseless aggression and violence

  - depression and risk of suicide $\uparrow \times 4$
  - schizophreniform psychosis (controversial associations)

  *n*ormal pre-morbid personality preserved
  *n*ice: warmer affect than in schizophrenia
  *n*egative family history of schizophrenia
  *n*eurological abnormalities $\uparrow$
  *n*ot distinguishable from schizophrenia on basis of psychopathology.

Neuropathology

11

DEMENTIAS

ALZHEIMER'S DISEASE (A. ALZHEIMER 1864–1915)

Macroscopic changes:

- shrunken gyri and widened sulci
- reduction of total brain weight (from in excess of 1200 g to less than 1000 g) because of symmetrical global cortical atrophy; greatest in medial temporal lobe especially parahippocampal gyrus (PHG)
- ventricular enlargement; greatest in temporal horns of lateral ventricles.

Microscopic changes:

- loss of pyramidal neurones from cortical layers III and V (especially younger patients)
- reduction of neurophil and synaptic innervation ($\downarrow$ synaptophysin and synapsin 1)
- neurofibrillary tangles (see below)
- amyloid plaques (see below)
- astrocyte proliferation
- granulovacuolar degeneration, especially in hippocampal pyramidal cells
- Hirano bodies.

- *Amyloid (neuritic/senile) plaques*: extracellular, insoluble core of beta-amyloid (A4 protein) fibrils (8 nm in diameter and 39–43 amino acids long) derived from amyloid precursor protein (APP), containing aluminium silicate and surrounded by degenerating neurites and astrocyte processes. Overall diameter up to 200 μm. Not specific to Alzheimer's disease (AD) (also found in normal ageing, Down's syndrome, Creutzfeldt–Jacob disease (CJD) and lead encephalopathy) but density correlates to severity of disease. APP gene is located on long arm of chromosome 21.
- *Neurofibrillary tangles (NFTs)*: intraneuronal, necessary for histological diagnosis and numbers correlate to severity of illness. Less common in non-dements but can occur in normal ageing, Down's syndrome, progressive supranuclear palsy,

postencephalitic Parkinson's disease, sub-acute sclerosing panencephalitis and dementia pugilistica.

- NFTs contain both straight filaments and paired helical filaments (PHFs). Abnormal phosphorylation of microtubular-associated protein (MAP) tau, produces paired helical filament-tau (double-helix PHF-tau). Phosphorylated tau – 68 kD molecular weight and also called A68 protein, Alzheimer's disease-associated protein (ADAP).
- Tau proteins associate with tubulin and alter cell shape. They are concentrated in neuronal axons.

- *Neurochemistry*: loss of basal forebrain (nucleus basalis of Meynert, medial septal nuclei and diagonal band of Broca) cholinergic cortical and hippocampal innervation
  - reduction in choline acetyl-transferase (ChAT) and acetylcholinesterase (AChE)
  - pre-synaptic nicotinic receptor concentration is reduced. Muscarinic M1 receptor activity is normal
  - reduced adrenergic and serotonergic cortical innervation:

    $\downarrow$ 5-HT$_2$ receptors in cortex (frontal, temporal, parietal) and hippocampus. Numbers of 5-HT$_2$ receptors and tangles inversely correlated and reduction of receptors is thought to be due to pyramidal cell loss
    $\downarrow$ α_2 adrenoceptors in hippocampus (α_1 receptors unchanged and α adrenoceptors unaltered in frontal and temporal cortices)
    $\downarrow$ β_1 receptors and $\uparrow$ β_2 receptors in prefrontal cortex along with reduction of NA

  - interneurone GABA levels are reduced (cortical loss of GABA reuptake markers)
  - cortical and hippocampal glutamate is reduced
  - somatostatin (co-localizes with GABA) is reduced
  - substance P, vasoactive intestinal peptide (VIP) and cholecystokinin (CCK) show no consistent changes
  - activity of second messenger systems adenylate cyclase (G$_s$-linked) and phophoinositide is reduced in frontal cortex of AD patients.

NON-ALZHEIMER DEMENTIAS

VASCULAR DEMENTIA

MULTI-INFARCT DEMENTIA

- *Macroscopic changes*:
  - localized/general brain atrophy
  - major vessel arteriosclerosis
  - ventricular enlargement
  - cerebral infarction* (cortical, subcortical, both) (infarction of specific brain regions, e.g. hippocampus or thalamus can in itself lead to dementia syndrome)
  - leukoaraiosis† (white matter rarefaction) (usually seen on CT scan or MRI).

*it is of note that there is usually no detectable cognitive impairment until 50 ml of brain tissue is affected, and usually dementia ensues once the area affected exceeds 100 ml. Also left hemisphere lesions more likely to be associated with clinical dementia.

†not specific for vascular dementias; found in 40 per cent of normal elderly population.

- *Microscopic changes*:
  - cell changes of ischaemic infarction.

BINSWANGER DISEASE (SUBACUTE ARTERIOSCLEROTIC ENCEPHALOPATHY) (O. BINSWANGER 1852–1929)

- *Macroscopic changes*:
  - lacunes
  - subcortical white matter demyelination
  - major vessel arteriosclerosis
  - neuronal loss
  - etat crible
  - ventricular enlargement.
- *Microscopic changes*:
  - gliosis.

CONGOPHILIC (AMYLOID) ANGIOPATHY

- *Macroscopic and microscopic changes*:
  - rare form of cerebral vessel specific amyloidosis with dominant inheritance. Associated with amyloid precursor protein gene mutation (Dutch family studies)
  - amyloid deposits (AD) in cerebral blood vessels cause weakening and predispose to lobar intracerebral haemorrhages or can cause narrowing of vessels and stenosis leading to ischaemia.

(NB Cerebral vessel amyloid deposition is seen in normal ageing and in up to 40 per cent of AD.)

LEWY BODY DEMENTIA

Lewy body: consists of dense core vesicles, MAP, tau protein, ubiquitin and protein neurofilaments.

Diffuse lewy body disease

- *Microscopic changes*:
  - subcortical Lewy bodies
  - neuronal loss from subcortical nuclei – basal nucleus of Meynert, substantia nigra, locus coeruleus
  - cortical Lewy bodies*
  - senile plaques
  - neurofibrillary tangles
  - reduced cortical choline acetyl transferase (CAT).

*temporal cortex, cingulate gyrus and parahippocampal gyrus particularly high content when compared to Lewy body concentrations in Parkinson's disease.

FRONTAL LOBE DEMENTIAS

PICK'S DISEASE (A. PICK 1851–1924)

- *Macroscopic changes*:
  - mild generalized atrophy
  - marked asymmetrical fronto-temporal atrophy (sparing of posterior one-third superior temporal gyrus)
  - affects white and grey matter leading to characteristic brownish 'knife-blade' gyri with spongiform change (grey/white boundary is blurred and white matter has rubbery consistency)
  - occasional atrophy of caudate and putamen
  - ventricular enlargement.
- *Microscopic changes* (observed in cortex, basal ganglia, substantia nigra, locus coeruleus):
  - severe neuronal loss (particularly outer cortical layers)
  - proliferation of astrocytes
  - fibrous gliosis
  - Pick cells (swollen cortical pyramidal cells also called balloon cells)*
  - Pick's bodies (intraneuronal argyrophilic inclusions)*.

(*present in up to one-third of cases. NB occasional distinction between Pick's disease (that with Pick cells and bodies) and frontal-lobe dementia (cases without these features). Distinction of limited use clinically.)
(NB plaques, tangles and Lewy bodies absent.)

SUBCORTICAL AND DEGENERATIVE DEMENTIAS

PROGRESSIVE SUPRANUCLEAR PALSY

Slow dementing syndrome with prominent neurological signs of unknown aetiology occurring in late adult life.

- *Macroscopic and microscopic changes:*
  - neuronal loss
  - subcortical and brainstem tangles (consisting of straight filaments).

  Huntington's disease
  Wilson's disease
  Hellervorden–Spatz disease (Martha–Alma disease) Rare recessive illness characterized by iron deposition in substantia nigra and globus pallidus.

- *Macroscopic changes:*
  - hypodensities seen on MRI scanning.
- *Microscopic changes:*
  - sea-blue histiocytes.

PRION DISEASES – ALTERED PRION PROTEINS (PrPᶜ)

CREUTZFELDT–JAKOB DISEASE

- *Macroscopic changes*:
    - brain atrophy is minimal if it occurs at all
    - can affect whole of CNS (especially spinal cord long descending tracts and anterior horn cells).
- *Microscopic changes*:
    - astrocyte proliferation
    - status spongiosus (cortical grey matter, basal ganglia, motor nuclei and thalamus)
    - neuronal degeneration and gliosis (without inflammation)
    - protease-resistant prion protein (PrPˢᶜ) accumulates in neurones and forms plaques.

GERSTMANN–STRAUSSLER–SCHEINKER SYNDROME (SPINOCEREBELLAR ATAXIA)

- *Microscopic changes*:
    - deposits akin to AD plaques containing scrapie amyloid protein.

PUNCH-DRUNK SYNDROME (BOXING ENCEPHALOPATHY)

- *Macroscopic changes*:
    - ventricular enlargement
    - corpus callosum thinning
    - cerebral atrophy
    - septum pellucidum perforation.
- *Microscopic changes*:
    - neuronal degeneration
    - neurofibrillary tangles.

CEREBRAL TUMOURS

1:20 000 in UK.

Second most common cause of cancer-related death in children less than 14 years of age.

- 80 per cent primary cerebral tumours (make up 10 per cent of all neoplasms);
    - 50 per cent derived from neuroepithelial cells:
        gliomas (see below)
        primitive neuro-ectodermal tumours (medulloblastoma, neuroblastoma)
        lymphoid tumours
    - 25 per cent mesodermal derivation
        menigiomas (often calcify)
        meningial sarcomas

– remainder:
> ectodermal derivation (pituitary adenoma, craniopharyngioma) vascular tissue derivatives (haemangioblastomas) neurilemmomas (Schwannomas), Schwann cell derivatives.
> (70 per cent of primary cerebral tumours: supratentorial in adults; *infra*-tentorial in *inf*ants and children (<14 years of age.))

- 20 per cent secondary, metastases: primary tumour in – lung, breast, kidney, colon, ovary and prostate.

Gliomas: derived from glial cells

- *astrocytomas*: commonest, grow diffusely, poorly encapsulated and graded I–IV. Grade IV (glioblastoma multiforme), most severe, has 3-year survival rate of 4 per cent
- *oligodendrogliomas*: slow growth, often calcify
- *ependymomas*: slow growing in ventricular system and can be intracranial or spinal.

Effects of cerebral tumours:

- *local*: focal signs – because of infiltration and destruction of tissue. May compromise circulation and cause oedema seizures: in about a third of cases, particularly if frontal or temporal lobes involved
- *generalized*: raised intracranial pressure (ICP).

RAISED INTRACRANIAL PRESSURE (ICP)

Mechanisms:

- ↑ brain volume
- space-occupying lesion
- oedema: cytotoxic (toxins and hyposia)
- vasogenic (excess extracellular fluid)
- ↑ cerebrospinal fluid (CSF)
- obstruction of flow at any level
- ↑ intracranial blood volume
- hypoxia
- hypercapnia
- trauma.

Signs and symptoms of ↑ ICP:

- *headache*: worst in mornings; exacerbated by coughing, sneezing, stooping and caused by deformation of dura and blood vessels
- *vomiting*: upon waking
- *papilloedema*: subarachnoid space extends along optic nerve
- *brain herniation*: subfalcine; transtentorial; produce false localizing signs
- *rostrocaudal migration of brainstem*: divided into stages. Diencephalic, mesencephalic, pontine and medullary reflects the progressive occlusion of brainstem blood vessels. At first the patient becomes drowsy, slipping into an unconscious

state and assuming a decerebrate posture. Blood pressure is raised and the heart rate falls (Cushing response). Pupils are initially dilated and fixed to light becoming **p**inpoint during the **p**ontine stage when the corneal reflexes are also lost. In the medullary stage the heart rate increases (tachycardia) and the blood pressure now falls. Respiration assumes a Cheyne–Stokes pattern and cardiac arrest is imminent.

(NB phenomenon of intracranial compliance – ICP increases can be buffered by displacement of CSF and blood.)

SCHIZOPHRENIA

Macroscopic and microscopic neuropathology from post-mortem and histological studies and structural and functional neuroimaging:

- ↓ brain mass and length
- ↓ cerebral grey matter volume (5–10 per cent reduction); especially temporal lobe; superior temporal gyrus is smaller particularly on left side
- ↓ size of cingulate and parahippocampal gyri
- ↓ size of hippocampus and amygdala (> on left)
- ↑ size of septum pellucidum with greater incidence of cavum septum pellucidum
- ↓ hippocampal neuronal size and mossy cell fibre staining displacement of pre-alpha and pre-beta-cells in entorhinal cortex
- ↓ neuronal density in anterior cingulate, primary motor and prefrontal cortices and thalamic medial dorsal nucleus, the cerebellum and nucleus accumbens
- no significant gliosis.

DEPRESSION

Neurotransmitter and receptor changes:

- ↓ noradrenergic function in depressives
- ↓ growth hormone response to clonidine (post-synaptic NA receptor down-regulation)
- ↓ CSF 3-methoxy-4-hydroxyphenylglycol (MHPG)
- ↓ platelet cAMP turnover (with clonidine stimulation).

Serotonergic function in depressives:

- ↓ plasma tryptophan (NB tryptophan depletion of recovered depressives continuing treatment causes temporary relapse)
- ↑ platelet 5-HT uptake presynaptically
- ↓ platelet imipramine binding 5-HT$_2$ post-synaptically
- ↓ CSF 5-HIAA (more so in those with a history of suicide and particularly those using violent methods) (NB thought to be associated with impulsive behaviour and also found in schizophrenia and personality disorders)
- ↓ cortisol response to ipsapirone challenge.

BIPOLAR DISORDER

Dopamine overactivity in mania.

NEUROPATHOLOGY OF CHRONIC ALCOHOL ABUSE

- *Seizures*: (10 per cent of alcoholics) due to:
  - direct toxicity of alcohol
  - head injury
  - withdrawal
  - hypoglycaemia.
- *Peripheral neuropathy*: (10 per cent) because of thiamine (B1) deficiency.
- *Cerebellar degeneration*: affects vermis and causes gait disturbance.
- *Wernicke–Korsakoff syndrome*: acute and chronic degenerative changes; caused by petechial haemorrhage, parenchymal degeneration and capillary proliferation of grey matter surrounding II and IV ventricles. (Mamillary bodies, hypothalamus, thalamus (dorso-medial nucleus), periaqueductal grey).
- *Optic atrophy*: because of vitamin B deficiency, associated heavy smoking, consumption of methanol.
- *Central pontine myelinolysis*: progressive demyelination of pontine (central) structures. Pseudobulbar palsy and spasticity.
- *Marchiafava–Bignami disease*: (especially red wine) demyelination of corpus callosum, cerebellar peduncles, optic tracts and cerebral hemisphere white matter. Leads to cognitive impairment, dementia, emotional lability, fits.
- *Myopathy*: (particularly proximal).

Neurophysiology

(see Figure 12.1)

The neuronal cell membrane has differential permeabilities that help create a negative **resting membrane potential** of $-70\,\text{mV}$. This is essential for neuronal function (**excitability**). The resting membrane potential is closer to the **equilibrium potential** (balance of electrical potential and concentration gradient) of K^+ ($-90\,\text{mV}$) than Na^+, as the resting membrane is more permeable to K^+. The **Na^+–K^+ ATPase pump** actively transports cations across the neuronal membrane ($3Na^+$ out for every $2K^+$ in), making a small direct contribution to the membrane potential because of this

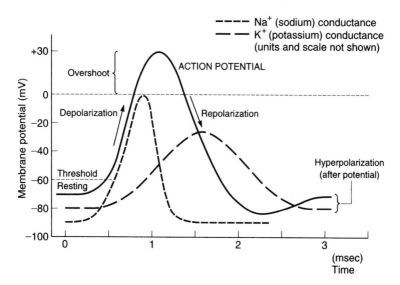

Figure 12.1 Action potential

outward transfer of cations, and a more significant indirect contribution by maintaining the ion concentration gradients.

Action potentials (AP) are rapid changes in the membrane potential involving transient (approx. 1 ms) local depolarization and repolarization. An AP can be:

- spontaneous (pacemaker activity)
- in response to activation of receptors
- because of synaptic stimulation.

NB transmission along axons is electrical, that across synapses is chemical.

The AP begins with rapid depolarization. During this 0.2–0.5 ms phase the permeability to Na^+ increases by a factor of 600 (activation) with initially insignificant change in K^+ permeability which lags behind. Na^+ ions therefore enter the neurone causing further depolarization and the membrane potential tends towards the equilibrium potential of Na^+ ($+60$ mV). Transiently the membrane polarity is reversed resulting in an 'overshoot'. Na^+ permeability is then inactivated and simultaneously K^+ permeability increases. Na^+ inactivation and the efflux of K^+ returns the membrane potential towards its resting value.

(NB the actual numbers of ions involved is extremely small and there is no change in the concentration gradients across the neuronal membrane during an AP.)

A typical AP lasts 1 ms. It is divided into several components.

To elicit an AP the membrane must depolarize beyond a critical level (threshold potential). For a typical neurone the threshold potential may be -60 mV and a stimulus that fails to depolarize the membrane to this level cannot elicit an AP. (NB axon hillock has lowest critical threshold.) However, an adequate stimulus can also fail to elicit an AP if the membrane is in its refractory period having been recently stimulated. The refractory period consists of an **absolute refractory period** (1 ms) (**ARP**) during which, regardless of stimulus strength, an AP cannot be elicited, and a **relative refractory period** (10 ms) (**RRP**) in which a very large stimulus may be able to elicit an AP. The ARP corresponds to Na^+ inactivation. The RRP corresponds to after hyperpolarization.

The propagation of an AP involves repeated axonal depolarization. Its velocity is dependent upon axonal diameter and myelination.

As diameter ↑ so velocity ↑. Myelination insulates membrane changes and causes APs to occur only at points of unmyelinated axon (**nodes of Ranvier**), resulting in **saltatory conduction**. Conduction velocities range from $1–100$ ms^{-1}.

Nerve fibres are classified by a variety of conventions (Tables 12.1, 12.2):

Table 12.1 Classification of nerve fibres

Nerve fibres	Diameter (μm)	Conduction velocity ms^{-1}	Function
A (α)	12–20	70–120	Motor somatic; proprioception
A (β)	5–12	30–70	Touch; pressure; kinaesthesia
A (γ)	3–7	15–30	Touch; pressure; motor
A (δ)	1–5	12–30	Pain; pressure; temperature
B	1–3	3–15	Preganglionic (autonomic)
C	up to 1	<2	Pain
C	up to 1	<2	Postganglionic (sympathetic)

Table 12.2 Alternative classification of nerve fibres

Nerve fibres	Diameter (μm)	Conduction velocity ms⁻¹	Function
Ia	12	70–120	Muscle spindle afferents
Ib			Tendon organs
II	10	25–70	Skin mechanoreceptors
III	3	10–25	Muscle deep pressure sensors
IV	1	1	Pain fibres (unmyelinated)

SYNAPSE (see Figure 12.2)

Specialized junction between two neurones (NB synapse with muscle–neuromuscular junction or plate).
Usually involves:

axon	and	dendrites	(axodendritic) but can involve
axon		cell body	(axonsomatic)
axon		axon	(axoaxonal)
dendrite		dendrite	(dendrodentritic)

The neurones involved are called **pre-synaptic** or **post-synaptic** depending on whether they carry APs towards or away from the synapse. Functionally synapses are of two types. Most synapses are chemical and rely on pre-synaptic release of neurotransmitters. Electrical synapses have direct membranous contact at **gap junctions** and transmit information faster than chemical synapses. **Conjoint synapses** have both chemical and electrical characteristics.

CHEMICAL SYNAPSE NEUROTRANSMISSION

The pre-synaptic neurone ends as a swelling called the **synaptic (terminal) bouton** or synaptic knob. This contains membrane-enclosed vesicles which store a chemical neurotransmitter. The pre-synaptic neurone is separated from the post-synaptic neurone by a **synaptic cleft** (200 Angstroms). The arrival of a pre-synaptic AP causes Ca^{2+} influx which initiates and assists pre-synaptic vesicle migration and fusion leading to synaptic cleft neurotransmitter release. The neurotransmitter diffuses across the synaptic cleft to combine with post-synaptic receptors. Neurotransmitter binding results in post-synaptic membrane permeability changes. The whole process takes 1 ms to occur and this is called the synaptic delay. Neurotransmitter inactivation terminates synaptic activity.

Synapses can be excitatory or inhibitory depending upon the characteristics of the neurotransmitter. An excitatory post-synaptic potential (EPSP) causes depolarization while an inhibitory post-synaptic potential (IPSP) causes hyperpolarization. EPSPs and IPSPs are electrotonic potentials (amplitude diminishes with increasing distance from site of initiation) and can be summated. This integration is necessary as a single EPSP (of 1 mV) is insufficient to reach an AP threshold. Potentials can combine temporally (temporal summation) and spatially (spatial summation). However, repeated stimulation at some synapses can result in diminishing post-synaptic potentials.

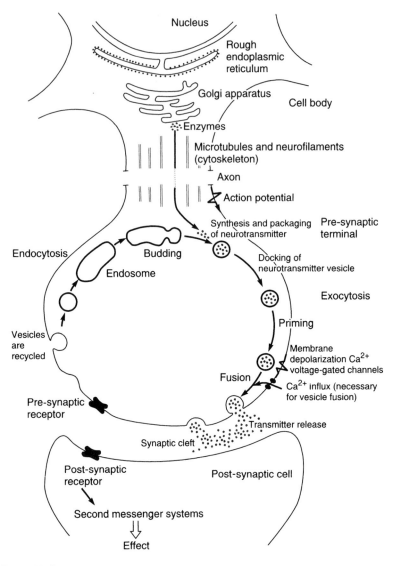

Figure 12.2 Synapse

This is called **post-tetanic depression**. Partial restriction of calcium influx augments the potentials, called **post-tetanic facilitation**, following which there is a brief increase in the size of the response called **post-tetanic potentiation**. Hippocampal post-tetanic potentiation can last several hours and is called **long-term potentiation (LTP)**. LTP involves L-glutamate and is associated with memory.

Synapses are unidirectional and ensure that APs (which propagate in both directions along the membrane) result in one-way neurotransmission along nerve fibres.

PERIPHERAL RECEPTORS

Receptors sense the external and internal environments. The sensory elements presented to receptors determine their characteristics and they are named accordingly.

Almost all receptors can be activated by more than one form of stimulus. However, they are specifically more sensitive to one kind of stimulus.

- *Exteroceptors*: e.g. receptors in skin sense immediate environment.
- *Telereceptors*: e.g. eyes and ears sense distant environment.
- *Nociceptors*: receptive to pain.
- *Thermoreceptors*: receptive to temperature.
- *Mechanoreceptors*: sense vibration and touch.
- *Proprioceptors*: sense position.

Receptors can be specialized nerve endings or distinct cellular structures connected to nerves.

SKIN RECEPTORS

- *Pacinian corpuscle*: pressure
- *Free nerve ending*: pressure, touch, pain, temperature
- *Merkel's disk*: pressure, touch
- *Peritrichial arborization*: pressure, touch
- *Meissner's corpuscle*: touch, discrimination
- *Ruffini ending*: pressure, touch, temperature
- *Krause's corpuscle*: temperature.

In mechanoreceptors such as the Pacinian corpuscle receptor activation results in an initial depolarization called the **generator potential (GP)**. This is very different from an AP (see Table 12.3).

Table 12.3 Action and generator potentials

	Action potential	Generator potentials
Duration (ms)	1–2	1–2
Refractory period	Yes (ARP 1 ms)	No
Conduction	Active; no loss of amplitude	Passive; amplitude decreases
Summation	No	Yes
Response	All-or-none	Graded

GP amplitude determines AP frequency only.
GP amplitude varies according to:

- intensity of stimulus
- its rate of change in application
- adaptation
- summation.

Thus sensory transduction is amplitude dependent, whereas transmission of information is frequency coded. Subsequent processing of sensory information includes

lateral inhibition, which allows the introduction of contrast by restricting the lateral spread of a stimulus amongst parallel inputs.

Adaptation is the reduction in AP frequency despite continuing stimulation. It occurs in both phasic and tonic receptors.

An increase in intensity of a stimulus can be coded by increased AP frequency and by activation of additional receptors/neurones. This is called **recruitment**.

MOTOR REFLEXES

MOTOR UNIT

Comprises a motor neurone axon and the muscle fibres it supplies. The innervation ratio (muscle fibres: innervating axons) which varies (4 in eye muscles; up to 2000 in postural muscles) determines the degree of muscular control. The force of contraction of a muscle is increased by increasing recruitment of motor units and then their discharge frequency.

STRETCH REFLEX (MYOSTATIC)

Stretch receptors called muscle spindles lie parallel to muscle fibres and are activated by lengthening of muscles. Annulospiral (primary) endings connect directly via Ia afferents to motor neurones and when stimulated cause contraction of the muscle. Important in tone/posture and movement.

Intrafusal muscle spindle → 1a neurones → spinal cord → extrafusal and motor neurone.

CLASP-KNIFE REFLEX (INHIBITORY)

Golgi tendon organs respond to muscle contraction and inhibit via Ib afferents to motor neurones further muscle contraction. Important in protecting and controlling muscular tension.

Golgi tendon organs → 1b neurones → spinal cord → α motor neurone inhibition.

SLEEP

Function: no clear theory has emerged – several possibilities:

- restoration and recovery (psychological and physical)
- consolidation of memories
- conservation of energy
- neural growth and repair
- resetting of emotions.

Definition: recurrent, regular, reversible state characterized by quiescence and diminished responsiveness to external stimuli.

The electroencephalogram (EEG) in an awake individual is random and fast. When resting quietly, with eyes closed, the EEG shows alpha waves. Muscle tone, measured by electromyogram (EMG) activity, is high and eye movements are present. The transition through drowsiness from being awake to sleeping is called the **hypnagogic period** and during this muscle tone diminishes, the eyes begin to roll and EEG alpha activity decreases.

Sleep is divided into **REM (rapid eye movement)** and non-REM sleep (see Table 12.4). REM sleep is also called desynchronized sleep and dreaming sleep.

Table 12.4 Difference between REM and non-REM sleep

	REM	Non-REM
Autonomic activity	Sympathetic	Parasympathetic
Heart rate	↑	↓
Blood pressure	↑	↓
Cerebral blood flow	↑	↓
Respiratory rate	↑	↓
Dreaming	↑	↓
Erection (penis)	Yes	–
Myoclonic jerks	Yes	–
Muscular tone	↓↓	↓
Ocular movements	Yes	Few

The normal pattern of sleep involves 4–5 cycles of alternating REM and non-REM sleep with REM sleep becoming progressively more prominent. The total time spent in REM sleep is 90 minutes in adults (20 per cent of total sleep period).

Other than brief periods of wakefulness (5 per cent of total sleep period) the remaining time is spent in non-REM sleep (75 per cent).

NON-REM SLEEP

Consists of four stages (after Rechtschaffen akales):

- *Stage 1* (5 per cent): As the individual falls asleep alpha activity diminishes to less than 50 per cent of the EEG record, giving way to characteristic low-amplitude, low-voltage **theta** activity. Occasional vertex sharp waves (V waves) are normal. EMG activity decreases and rolling eye movements are present.
- *Stage 2* (55 per cent): Now in light sleep the EEG shows low-voltage, slow frequencies (theta waves) that are interrupted intermittently by **K complexes** and **sleep spindles**. The latter are spindle-shaped EEG traces of short bursts (0.5 s) of waves (12–14 Hz). K complexes are high-voltage spikes consisting of a negative wave followed 0.75 s later by a positive wave.
- *Stage 3* (5 per cent): The onset of deep sleep is accompanied by the appearance on EEG of high amplitude (75 μV), low frequency (2 Hz) **delta waves**, which by definition form less than 50 per cent but more than 20 per cent of the trace.
- *Stage 4* (10 per cent): Delta waves form more than **50 per cent** of EEG activity. Collectively stages 3 and 4 are called **slow wave sleep** or **synchronized sleep**. Sleep spindles can occur in slow wave sleep.

REM SLEEP

The EEG in REM sleep is characterized by random, fast mixed-frequency activity of low voltage (similar to awake state), hence it is also called **paradoxical sleep**. It is distinguished by **saw-tooth waves**.

Sleep can be plotted as a **hypnogram**. In a normal adult the pattern of sleep is as follows:

after entering sleep the individual progresses through stages 1–4 and then returns to stage 3 and then 2. From stage 2, having been asleep for about 90 minutes, the individual enters their first period of REM sleep. The individual then reverts to stage 2 sleep and the cycle is repeated 4–5 times during the night with each cycle lasting 90 minutes. As sleep progresses the proportion of REM sleep increases and that of slow-wave sleep decreases.

SLEEP CHANGES WITH AGE

Newborn sleeps 16 hours a day and is able to pass directly from wakefulness into REM sleep, which takes up more than 50 per cent of sleep. By 4 months REM forms 40 per cent of total sleep and is usually preceded by non-REM sleep.

Continuity of sleep is greatest in early childhood. It is least at extremes of age.

A young adult sleeps 8 hours a day of which 90 minutes (approx. 20 per cent) is REM sleep.

NEUROCHEMICAL CORRELATES OF SLEEP

• Sleep is promoted by – ACh(REM), GABA.
• Sleep is inhibited by – Noradrenaline, 5-HT, Dopamine, Histamine.

NEUROENDOCRINE CORRELATES OF SLEEP

As sleep *sTarTs* – *T*estosterone levels ↑
*P*rolactin *P*eaks *P*rior to waking (↑ last two hours of sleep)
REM sleep – ↓ *RE*nin and ↓ *M*elatonin
*S*low-wave *S*leep – peaks of *S*omato*S*tain (SS)
Growth *H*ormone levels – High
Cortiso*l* levels – Low

SLEEP–WAKE CYCLE

Two main theories:

1 **Cellular (Hobson's) model** Involves three groups of central neurones:
   – nucleus reticularis pontis caudalis (gigantocellular tegmental field of pons) cholinergic neurones function as 'on' cells promoting REM sleep.

– dorsal raphe nuclei serotonergic neurones and locus coeruleus noradrenergic neurones function as 'off' cells and a gradual increase in their activity inhibits the REM-promoting cholinergic cells and allows slow-wave sleep to resume.
– there is little support for this model.

2 **Monoaminergic (Jouvet's, two-stage or biochemical) model**
   – slow-wave sleep (non-REM) is associated with Raphe complex serotonergic neuronal activity. Destruction of these neurones leads to insomnia. Serotonin precursor tryptophan is hypnotic.
   – locus coeruleus noradrenergic neuronal activity associated with REM sleep. Destruction leads to selective REM suppression.

Lesion effects Elimination of all somatosensory inputs by sectioning below medulla (encephale isole) preserves normal sleep–wake cycle.
   Mid-pontine transection leads to being permanently awake.
   Mid-collicular brainstem transection leads to permanent sleep.
   Hence *a*rousal *a*rea *a*bove sleep-promoting area.

EEG

In 1929 Hans Berger first described electroencephalography as a safe means of investigating brain function. The standard electroencephalogram (EEG) involves recording from electrodes placed on the scalp according to the international 10–20 system.

Normally 40 electrodes are applied using the nasion, inion and left and right auricular depressions as landmarks, and recording is done from 8 or 16 channels.

A standard EEG recording includes:

• several minutes at rest (and perhaps BLeep)
• whilst overbreathing (hyperventilation)
• during exposure to flashing lights (photic stimulation).

Activating procedures provoke abnormalities.
   The normal activity range is 1–40 Hz frequency and 5–150 μV amplitude.
   EEG is useful in diagnosing, defining and monitoring the treatment of epilepsy.
   However, a *no*rmal EEG does *no*t exclude epilepsy.
   Specialized forms of recording allow measurement of activity from specific parts of the brain e.g. nasopharyngeal and sphenoidal recordings detect medial temporal lobe activity (see Table 12.5).

Table 12.5

Type of recording	Electrode placement
Sphenoidal	Between zygoma and mandibular coronoid notch
Nasopharyngeal	Superior nasopharynx
Electrocorticography	Surface of the brain
Depth electroencephalography	Inside the brain

Other means of recording the EEG:

- ambulatory EEG – record is maintained on suitable portable recorder
- video and event recorders can be used to correlate clinical findings with those of EEG
- telemetric recording provides a record from a distance.

Normal EEG wave patterns: (classified according to frequency Hz)
BATHED

Table 12.6

Wave type	Frequency (Hz)
*B*eta:	>13
*A*lpha:	8–13
*THE*ta:	4–8
*D*elta:	<4

- *Beta activity (β)*: awake resting adult with open eyes. Activity is related to sensory-motor cortical stimulation and is enhanced by anxiety. Best recorded from fronto-central positions. Variance according to cortical site described as **desynchronization** (simultaneous waves are out of phase). Beta displacement of alpha activity upon arousal is called **alerting** or **arousal response** and described as **alpha blocking**.
- *Alpha activity (α)*: awake resting adult EEG pattern that is most prominent over the occipital region. It is accentuated by eye closure and attenuated by attention. It has a circadian rhythm and varies according to menstrual cycle. Amplitude can be attenuated by a fall in temperature and augmented by an increase. Its frequency diminishes with age and an inter-hemispheric difference of 1 Hz is pathological.
- *Theta activity (θ)*: unusual in waking adult (found transiently in 15 per cent of individuals). Normal in children aged 2–5 years and can be evoked by frustration. Also found in psychopaths.
- *Delta activity (δ)*: abnormal in waking adult, may signify brain neoplasm. Characteristic of deep sleep and common in children, particularly infants. Induced by overbreathing. Diffuse cortical distribution.
- *Lambda activity (λ)*: single, occipital sharp waves associated with ocular movements during visual scanning (associated with *l*ooking).
- *Mu activity (μ)*: arch-like waves that occur over precentral (*m*otor) cortex. Related to *m*ovement and mitigated by motion of contralateral limb.
- *V waves*: normal phenomenon of sharp electronegative waves that occur over the vertex in response to an auditory stimulus. Also seen in drowsiness.
- *Spikes*: brief peaks of less than 80 ms duration.
- *Sharp waves*: prominent wave formations of 80–200 ms duration.

EEG variance with age:

- full-term *n*ew-born EEG activity is almost *n*il
- infant (<1 year) EEG desynchronized delta activity
- *t*oddler (>2 years) EEG *t*heta activity predominates
- *a*dolescent (second decade of life) EEG *a*lpha activity is established
- *a*geing adult *a*lpha activity *a*ttenuates in *a*mplitude and frequency
- focal anterior temporal delta activity occurs in third of those over 60 years.

Activating procedures: used to elicit EEG abnormalities not discernible in standard EEG:

- hyperventilation: cerebral hypoxia → cortical hyperexcitability
- photic stimulation (photic driving): (20–30 Hz) synchronizes alpha rhythm
- sleep deprivation.

EEG CHANGES

May signify pathology and can sometimes be diagnostic (see below).
   Can be because of surgical interventions, ECT and medication.
   About 15 per cent of EEG abnormalities are false positives.

EEG artefacts can be caused by:

- muscular contraction (local)
- eye movement
- cardiac arrhythmias.

PATHOLOGY

Organic psychoses (haemorrhage, infarction, infection, trauma, metabolic or endocrine disorders):

- usually diffuse symmetrical changes: ↓ α and ↑ δ and θ
- focal lesions, e.g. tumours, subdural haematoma EEG changes asymmetrical

(NB non-organic stupor, e.g. because of depression or schizophrenia alpha activity is preserved).

Epilepsy:

- temporal lobe (TLE) sleep EEG + routine EEG detect spike foci in 90 per cent.
- petit mal: generalized compound waves and spikes with frequency of 3 Hz.

Dementias:

- Alzheimer's: 95 per cent of those with definite AD have abnormal EEG
- alpha activity decreases and delta/theta activity increases.
- multi-infarct dementia: EEG of little help.
- Pick's disease: 50 per cent have abnormal EEG. Alpha activity better preserved than in AD.

Infections:

- HIV – diffuse slowing.
- subacute sclerosing panencephalitis (SSP): bilateral, symmetrical and synchronous high amplitude polyphasic sharp wave and slow wave complexes in burst of up to **10 seconds** often accompanied by myoclonic jerks.
- Herpes simplex encephalitis: **1–3 seconds** repetitive episodic discharges along with temporal lobe focal slow waves.

   Creutzfeld–Jakob disease: bilateral, synchronous generalized irregular spike-wave complexes occurring at intervals of **0.5–1.0 seconds**, often accompanied by myoclonic jerks. EEG is always abnormal. (cf. Description of SSP above.)

Huntingdon's chorea: characteristic (not specific) diffuse flattening of EEG with low amplitude theta and delta waves.

Hepatic encephalopathy: triphasic waves and widespread slowing.

Hypoxia: occipital alpha rhythm is gradually replaced by theta and delta activity. Then with severe hypoxia there is initially intermittent cortical suppression resulting in a 'burst-suppression' effect which then progressively gives way to a flat EEG trace.

Midbrain tegmentum infarction: severe brainstem injury results in invariant alpha rhythm (alpha-coma).

Table 12.7   Medication and physical treatments

Change	Medications		
↑β	Barbiturates	Benzodiazepines	Tricyclic antidepressants (TCAs)
↑θ	Barbiturates	Benzodiazepines	TCAs Neuroleptics
↑δ			TCAs Neuroleptics

Alcohol increases *a*lpha activity. Delirium tremens – increased fast activity.

Carbamazepine increases slow-wave sleep (see Table 12.7).

Lithium may produce focal slow waves in proportion to concentration.

ECT – between treatments there is diffuse EEG slowing (frontal region slowest to recover) increasing with each treatment and normalizing one month post-ECT.

Psychosurgery – increased bi-frontal delta activity.

EVOKED POTENTIALS

Repeated stimulation of sensory modality results in neuronal, brainstem and cortical electrical responses which can only be discerned from background activity by signal averaging. Electrical responses are measured as evoked potentials (EP) typically consisting of a negative and positive component (negative upgoing and positive downgoing). Components are labelled according to their latency (time from stimulus to peak deflection) and direction of deflection: e.g. P100 – positive peak 100 ms after stimulus.

TYPES OF EVOKED POTENTIALS

VEPs (visual EP) – e.g. increase in latency of P100 on exposure to patterned stimulus (chess board) in individual with optic neuritis because of multiple sclerosis.

AEPs (auditory EP).

SEPs (somatosensory EP).

Following a stimulus:

- *Short potential* (<20 ms): corresponds to sensory pathway activity.
- *Late potential* (70–200 ms): cortical arrival and elaboration of sensory information.
- *Cognitive potential* (>200 ms): more complex processing of information, e.g. **P300**, an event-related potential (ERP), seen 300–500 ms following stimulation and possibly

relates to cognition and the formation of memory. P300 is maximal over parietal cortex regardless of sensory modality. It is altered in Down's syndrome, of diminished amplitude in autism, schizophrenia and Alzheimer's disease and larger in developmental dysphasia. The changes are not specific.

- *Contingent negative variation (CNV)*: like P300, is an event-related slow potential that is elicited by initially providing a priming stimulus and then one which requires a response. It is also called the **expectancy wave** and consists of a slow negative potential shift particularly in frontal areas and vertex. Correlates to attention and motivation and is therefore attenuated by lack of stimulation and drugs such as barbiturates.
- *Bereitschaftspotential (readiness potential)*: slow negative potential precedes voluntary movement by 1 second.

NOVEL TECHNIQUES

BRAIN ELECTRICAL ACTIVITY MAPPING (BEAM)

EEG or EP data presented as maps, allowing summation, averaging and statistical analysis of such information.

MAGNETOENCEPHALOGRAPHY (MEG)

Involves the measurement of magnetic fields created by brain electrical potentials. It is a type of functional imaging with very low latency.

Neurochemistry

13

Neurotransmitters are released at neuronal synapses whereupon they bind to specific receptors to produce specific responses. To be defined as a neurotransmitter it must be present in neuronal endings along with the necessary means for its synthesis and degradation.

Neurotransmitters are stored in pre-synaptic vesicles and released into the synaptic cleft in response to a stimulus. This is a Ca^{2+}-dependent process involving the fusion of neurotransmitter vesicles with specific pre-synaptic areas.

Of the neurotransmitters important to psychiatry, acetylcholine (ACh), serotonin (5-hydroxytryptamine, 5-HT) and the catecholamines noradrenaline (NA) and dopamine (DA) will be discussed in detail by illustrating their synthesis, degradation and actions. The amino-acids gamma-aminobutyric acid (GABA) and glutamate also have important neurotransmitter functions, as do some peptides (vasoactive intestinal peptide, endorphins, cholecystokinin, somatostatin, neurotensin).

ACETYLCHOLINE (see Figure 13.1)

Synthesis Acetylcholine (ACh) is synthesized in a single reaction:

$$\text{choline} + \text{acetyl CoA} \rightleftharpoons \text{acetylcholine} + \text{coenzyme A}$$

This is catalysed by **choline acetyltransferase (ChAT)** which is selective for cholinergic neurones in the nervous system. ChAT is synthesized in the rough endoplasmic reticulum of the perikaryon and taken via axoplasmic transport to the axon terminals where it is mostly free in the cytoplasm.

The rate of ACh synthesis is dependent upon the catalytic activity of ChAT, which in turn is primarily dependent upon the availability of choline. This ChAT is not in itself rate limiting. ChAT activity is altered by neuronal activity and is inhibited by ACh (product inhibition) through an allosteric ACh-binding site on the enzyme. When

ACh binds to ChAT it alters the three-dimensional conformation of the molecule and reduces its catalytic activity.

Choline is found in food such as vegetables, seeds, egg yolk and liver. It is also produced in the liver and transported across the blood–brain barrier (BBB) by a specific bi-directional carrier system situated in the endothelial cells of the capillaries. A low-affinity choline uptake mechanism exists in all cells and the choline is used for the synthesis of phospholipids.

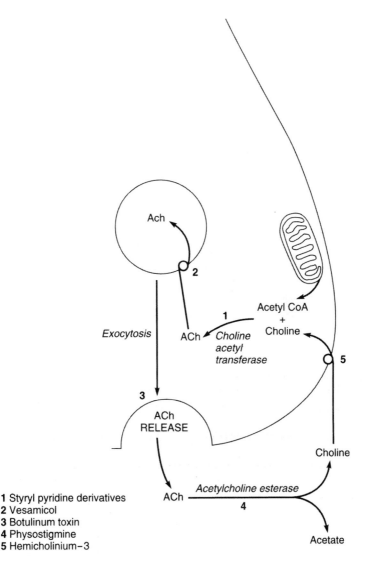

1 Styryl pyridine derivatives
2 Vesamicol
3 Botulinum toxin
4 Physostigmine
5 Hemicholinium–3

Figure 13.1 Cholinergic neurone

In the brain, choline is used for the synthesis of phosphatidylcholine and ACh. A large proportion of choline is recycled as it is retrieved following the degradation of ACh by a sodium-dependent, high-affinity, carrier-mediated mechanism that is specific to cholinergic neurones.

Coenzyme A contains adenine, a purine nucleotide base, and is found in mitochondria. Addition of an acetyl group to its sulphydryl group produces acetyl CoA.

Acetyl CoA is synthesized by the mitochondrial pyruvate dehydrogenase complex using pyruvate derived from glycolysis. Acetyl CoA is mainly used in the tricarboxylic acid cycle for the generation of energy, in the form of **ATP**. However, some is used for cytoplasmic ACh synthesis.

ACh storage/release: ACh is stored in vesicles that originate in the cell body. These are transported to the nerve terminals and after ACh release they are recycled. There are two populations of ACh vesicles:

- VP_1: reserve vesicles that are large and of low density
- VP_2: recycled vesicles that are small and dense.

ACh inactivation Two means:

- diffusion out of synaptic cleft
- degradation.

$$Ach + H_2O \rightarrow^* choline + acetic\ acid\ (^*cholinesterase)$$

Cholinesterases: acetylcholinesterase (AChE) and butyrylcholinesterase (BChE).

Both are found in both brain and muscle. BChE (pseudocholinesterase) is found in brain glial cells, blood and liver.

AChE has greater specificity for ACh and is found in cholinergic neurones. It is a glycoprotein with two binding sites (anionic and esteratic). ACh degradation is a two-stage process involving a transient unstable intermediate acetylated AChE, in which the enzyme is covalently bound via serine.

THE ACTION OF DRUGS

- ACh synthesis:
    - *hemicholinium-3 and triethylcholine*: inhibit high-affinity choline uptake. Choline and lecithin are acetyl precursors which increase turnover.
- ACh storage/release:
    - *vesamicol*: inhibits vesicular transport
    - *α-latrotoxin*: (venom of black widow spider) depletes vesicles
    - *clostridial neurotoxins*: botulinum/tetanus disrupt vesicle exocytosis.
    - *3,4 diaminpyridine and phosphatidylserine* promote ACh release.
- ACh mimetics:
    - *carbachol, pilocarpine and bethanechol* act on post-synaptic receptors (see Receptors page 147).
- ACh degradation:
    - *reversible/competitive anticholinesterases*
        edrophonium: used diagnostically (myasthenia gravis)
        physostigmine: treatment of glaucoma

neostigmine: does not cross BBB
long-acting **tacrine** and **donepazil** treatment of Alzheimer's disease
– *irreversible anticholinesterases*
malathion, parathion
nerve gases (sarin, tabun and di-isopropyl fluorophosphate).

CATECHOLAMINES (DOPAMINE, NORADRENALINE AND ADRENALINE)

Catecholamines are monoamines (dopamine, DA; noradrenaline, NA; and adrenaline, Ad) that possess the catechol group. DA, NA and Ad share a common synthetic pathway illustrated in Figures 13.2 and 13.3.

The rate-limiting enzyme in the synthetic pathway is **tyrosine hydroxylase** (TH). TH consists of four identical subunits and contains Fe^{2+} ions that are essential for its activity. Also necessary is the pteridine cofactor, tetrahydrobiopterin (THB_4). Catecholamine synthesis can be inhibited by inhibitors of TH. This can be achieved by:

* chelation of Fe^{2+} ions
* competitive inhibition at pteridine-binding site
* competitive inhibition at tyrosine-binding site.

α-**methyl-para-tyrosine (AMPT)** binds at tyrosine-binding site to inhibit TH.

Note that progression from dopamine to NA and Ad is dependent upon having the necessary enzymes.

Both acute and long-term mechanisms are used to regulate TH.

Acute mechanisms:

* end-product inhibition (catecholamines inhibit TH)
* stimulation-induced activation: neural activity increases enzyme hydroxylation by increasing the maximum velocity of the reaction and decreasing the effect of end-product inhibition
* enzyme activation by phosphorylation of regulatory serine residues:
  – ser-19: Ca^{2+} and calmodulin-dependent protein kinase II (CaM-K II)
  – ser-31: extracellular signal-regulated kinases (ERKs)
  – ser-40: cAMP-dependent protein kinase
* substrate availability: only of importance at high rates of activity.

Long-term mechanism:

* *trans-synaptic induction*: following stressful stimuli (e.g. cold, reserpine depletion) TH gene transcription and synthesis is increased.

Catecholamine storage: prior to synaptic release, catecholamines are stored in vesicles. In addition to the catecholamine, other vesicular constituents are ascorbic acid, calcium, nucleotides, chromogranins and dopamine β-hydroxylase (DBH). The necessary proteins are synthesized in the smooth endoplasmic reticulum (smER) and transferred to the Golgi apparatus where they undergo post-translational modification (addition of sulphate, phosphate or carbohydrate groups). The vesicles form by budding from

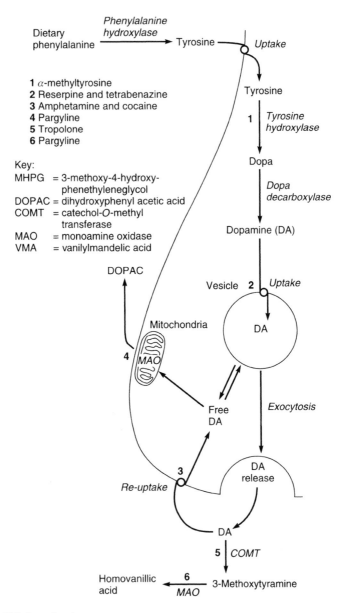

Figure 13.2 Dopaminergic neurone

the Golgi apparatus. ATP is transported into the vesicles, and cytoplasmic dopamine is actively taken up. Within the vesicle DA can then be converted to NA which can subsequently be converted to Ad in the cytoplasm. For this latter step, NA moves into the cytoplasm and, once converted, Ad is taken up by the vesicle.

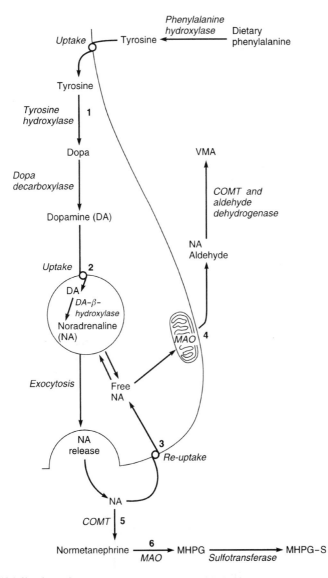

Figure 13.3 Noradrenergic neurone

The uptake of catecholamines into secretory vesicles is dependent upon a vesicular membrane proton-translocating ATPase which moves protons into the vesicle. This creates an intra-vesicular pH of ~5.5 and an electrical potential such that there is a combined electrochemical gradient favouring the movement of catecholamines into the vesicles.

The catecholamine transporters can be inhibited by **tetrabenazine** and **reserpine**.

Catecholamine release: catecholamine release follows Ca^{2+}-dependent exocytosis and occurs in response to stimulation (membrane depolarization), and can therefore be inhibited by **tetrodotoxin (TTX)** (blocks Na^+ channels). Catecholamine release is stimulated by **methylphenidate** and **amphetamine**.

Catecholamine inactivation: catecholamine effects are terminated by uptake and catabolism.

Synaptic uptake: Na^+Cl^--dependent co-transport of ions and catecholamines. Energy for this is derived from Na^+–K^+ ATPase and so uptake is inhibited by ouabain.

Synaptic uptake transporters for NA, DA, 5-HT, glutamate and GABA are glycoproteins with 12 transmembrane domains. Neuronal NA uptake is by uptake 1 and that into extra-neuronal tissues is by uptake 2. The two mechanisms differ.

Synaptic catecholamine uptake inhibitors:

amphetamine
cocaine*
mazindol*†
methylphenidate†
tricyclic antidepressants†

* also 5-HT transporter uptake inhibitors.
† greater activity at NA uptake transporter than DA transporter.

Catecholamine catabolism: involves two main enzymes: **monoamine oxidase (MAO)** and **catechol-O-methyltransferase (COMT)**.

MAO is found in the outer membrane of *m*itochondria in both neurones and glial cells (see Tables 13.1 and 13.2). Also found in liver and kidney cells. Requires flavin adenine dinulcleotide (FAD) as cofactor and catalyses oxidative deamination of monoamines. Two types MAO-A and -B:

Table 13.1

	MAO-A	MAO-B
Preferred substrates	NA, Ad, DA, 5-HT	β-Phenylethylamine, benzylamine, DA

MAO-B is found in platelets and its level is stable with time, though there is a tendency for these to increase with age.

Table 13.2 MAO inhibitors

Irreversible	Non-selective	Isocarboxacid	
		Pargyline	
		Tranylcypromine	
	Selective	Clorgyline	(MAO-A)
		Deprenyl	(MAO-B)
Reversible	Selective	Moclobemide	(MAO-A)

COMT is found in the synaptic cleft. It exists in both soluble and membrane-bound forms and it is also found in liver, kidney and heart cells. Brain COMT in soluble form is largely extra-neuronal (glial cells, ependymal cells, cells of choroid plexus).

The enzyme is Mg^{2+} dependent and catalyses the transfer of a methyl group from S-adenosyl-methionine (SAM) to a hydroxyl group of catechol compounds.

COMT is inhibited by **pyrogallol** and **tropolone**.

SEROTONIN

Serotonin synthesis Serotonin is an indolealkylamine (5-HT) neurotransmitter synthesized from tryptophan. The rate-limiting step in synthesis is catalysed by **tryptophan hydroxylase** (TrpH). This enzyme is specific to serotonergic neurones and therefore can also serve as a marker for 5-HT neurones.

TrpH is synthesized in the cell bodies and transported to the nerve terminals. It can be inhibited by **p-chlorophenylalanine** (PCPA), 6-fluorotryptophan and **p-chloroamphetamine** (PCA).

Table 13.3 Central serotonergic nuclei

N. raphe pallidus	N. raphe dorsalis
N. raphe obscuris	N. raphe pontis
N. raphe magnus	N. raphe centralis superior

Ascending fibres innervate the striatum, hypothalamus, amygdala (dorsal nuclei) and hippocampus (median raphe). Regulate sleep cycle, mood, appetite, libido and body temperature (see Table 13.3).

Descending fibres → dorsal horn of the spinal cord: inhibit pain transmission
→ ventral horn: regulate motor neuron output.

Serotonin storage and release (see Figure 13.4) 5-HT is stored in vesicles bound to serotonin-binding protein (SBP). It is released into the synapse following membrane depolarization induced calcium influx and exocytosis. **Fenfluramine** and **PCA** release serotonin.

Release is regulated by somatodendritic (5-HT_{1A}) and pre-synaptic (5-HT_{1B} and 5-HT_{1B}) autoreceptors that inhibit cell firing and 5-HT release respectively. Autoreceptor antagonists such as **pindolol** can therefore augment 5-HT release.

SEROTONIN INACTIVATION

Serotonin uptake: a carrier-mediated energy-dependent process. The 5-HT transporter belongs to a family of carrier proteins and has 12 transmembrane domains. 5-HT binds to the carrier in protonated form (5-HT^+) and is co-transported, with Na^+ and Cl^- ions, across the membrane and then returns bound to K^+.

Serotonin uptake is inhibited by tricyclic antidepressants (TCAs) such as imipramine and clomipramine and more selectively by 'selective serotonin re-uptake inhibitors' (SSRIs) such as citalopram, fluoxetine, fluvoxamine, paroxetine and sertraline. Inhibition of synaptic re-uptake increases the synaptic concentration of 5-HT.

Serotonin metabolism MAO metabolizes 5-HT by oxidative deamination. The resulting aldehyde is oxidized to 5-hydroxyindoleacetic acid (5-HIAA). 5-HIAA diffuses out of neurones into cerebrospinal fluid (CSF). 5-HIAA is removed from the CSF by the choroid plexus and this process is inhibited by **probenecid**.

EXCITATORY AMINO ACIDS (EAA)

Amino acids (aa): consist of an α-carbon atom that has four different chemical groups attached to it (exception glycine). Hence two stereoselective isomers denoted L and D

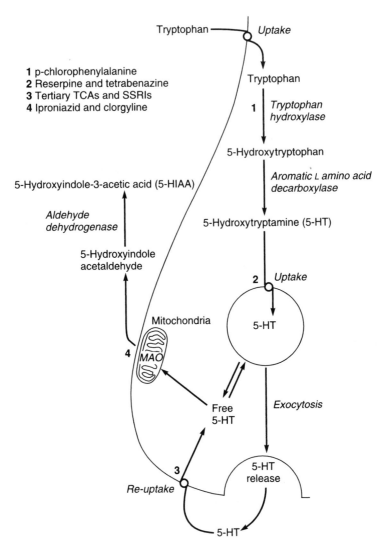

Figure 13.4 Serotonergic neurone

forms. L is aa's predominant form *in vivo*. At physiological pH aas are ionized and possess both negative and positive charges and are therefore known as **zwitterions**. If an aa side-chain has an amine group then it is likely to be a basic aa; if the side-chain has a carboxyl group then it is likely to be an acidic aa.

EAAs: glutamate is the principal EAA. Additionally there is some evidence supporting a similar more limited role for aspartate and possibly others such as cysteic acid and homocysteic acid.

GLUTAMATE

Glutamate is a non-essential aa that is synthesized by α-ketoglutarate (AKG) transamination. The enzyme alanine aminotransferase has pyridoxal phosphate as a cofactor and AKG is derived from the oxidative metabolism of glucose (glycolysis).

Glutamate is also synthesized from glutamine. Glutamine is stored in astrocytes and an ATP requiring mitochondrial enzyme, glutaminase, converts glutamine to glutamate.

$$\text{glutamine} + H_2O + ATP \rightarrow \text{glutamate} + ADP + NH_4^+ + PO_4^-$$

This reaction forms part of the glutamine cycle. In this glutamine is synthesized from glutamate catalyzed by glutamine synthetase. There is differential localization of substrates and enzymes in neuronal endings and neighbouring astrocyte processes.

Breakdown of glutamate can be by conversion to glutamine (as described), by transamination to AKG or by oxidative deamination to AKG by glutamate dehydrogenase.

Glutamate is a fast-acting neurotransmitter that is distributed widely and found in significant concentrations in the hippocampus, its projections and those of neocortical pyramidal cells, and also in cerebellar cortical parallel fibres. However, accurate functional localization is difficult because glutamate is a precursor to GABA and is an intermediary in metabolic processes.

INHIBITORY AMINO ACIDS (GABA AND GLYCINE)

GAMMA-AMINOBUTYRIC ACID (GABA)

GABA is widely distributed within the brain with highest density in the hypothalamus, basal ganglia, amygdala and limbic nuclei. It is synthesized via a single reaction catalyzed by glutamate decarboxylase. This enzyme which has pyridoxal phosphate as a cofactor converts L-glutamate to GABA within neuronal axon terminals.

GABA is metabolized by a mitochondrial enzyme, GABA aminotransferase, which converts it along with AKG to glutamate and succinic semialdehyde. The latter is converted to succinate and the metabolism of AKG to succinate in this manner is called the 'GABA shunt'.

* *Allylglycine*: inhibits glutamate decarboxylase.
* *Gamma-vinyl GABA (vigabatrin)* inhibits GABA aminotransferase.

Synaptic release of GABA from vesicular storage is by exocytosis and re-uptake is via GABA transporters, of which there are two types. Uptake can be inhibited by **nipecotic acid, β-alanine** and **2,4-diaminobutyric acid (DABA)**.

GLYCINE

Glycine is synthesized from serine in a single reaction catalysed by serine hydroxymethyltransferase which has tetrahydrofolate as a co-factor. It can also be synthesized by the transamination of glyoxylate derived from glycolysis or the TCA cycle. Glycine is metabolized to glutathione or guanidoacetic acid.

Synaptic release is by exocytosis and uptake is via sodium-dependent transporters of which there are three types (GlyT-1a, GlyT-1b and GlyT-2). GlyT-1a and 1b are found predominantly in grey and white matter respectively, while GlyT-2 is found in the cerebellum, brainstem and spinal cord. Spinal cord Renshaw cell motor neurone inhibition is glycine mediated and it plays an important role in both motor and sensory systems.

HISTAMINE

Histamine is a biogenic amine that is synthesized from histidine by decarboxylation (histidine decarboxylase). Peripherally it is found in mast cells and takes part in many inflammatory and allergic reactions. Histamine is found in the brain in histaminergic neurone cell bodies, situated mainly in the hypothalamus, mast cells, neurolipomastocytes and capillary endothelial cells. Histamine is often co-localized with GABA or neuropeptides. Following synaptic release there is no uptake and instead histamine is inactivated by enzymes histamine N-methyltransferase and MAO-B.

RECEPTORS

All recognized neurotransmitters have been found to have more than one type of receptor (receptor subtypes).

Receptor subtypes may be derived from common genes through gene duplication, mutation and recombination or via alternative mRNA splicing. Receptor subtypes confer neurotransmitters diversity of effect (e.g. excitation/inhibition through differing transduction mechanisms) and can be characterized pharmacologically and through gene cloning.

Neurotransmitter receptors (NtRs) belong to one of two families of membrane proteins:

1 **G-protein-coupled neurotransmitter receptors** (GP-NtRs) (**metabotropic receptors**) (action reliant on metabolic steps): consist of a single protein molecule with seven transmembrane regions (domains). Four of these domains form part of the extracellular NT-binding site and two intracellular regions of the protein form the G-protein-binding site. GP-NtRs are coupled to specific **G-proteins** which, once activated, stimulate membrane effectors. These are usually enzymes involved in **second messenger systems** which in turn mediate cellular responses. These types of NtRs are relatively slow to respond.
2 **Ligand-gated channels** (**ionotropic receptors**): consist of five subunits arranged in the membrane to provide an ion channel. The channel possesses an NT-binding site which acts as a gate. Subunit heterogeneity provides functional variety through differential specificity of different subunits. The ionic permeability of the channel determines its action. Receptor function can be further modulated through occupancy of **allosteric binding sites**. These types of NtRs are fast acting.

G-PROTEINS

Heterotrimers consisting of three subunits α, β and γ. There are several different kinds of each type of subunit (e.g. α_s, α_i, α_o, α_q). α subunits have a guanyl-binding site (GBS) for guanyl nucleotides (GDP and GTP) and determine overall G-protein specificity and designation (e.g. G_s proteins contain α_s subunits). G-proteins can only assume two functional conformations; GDP bound or GTP bound. When the G-protein is inactive GDP is bound to its GBS and all three subunits are associated forming a trimer. Agonist-stimulated receptor interaction leads to GTP substitution of GDP, and α subunit dissociation leaves behind a βγ dimer. The α subunit and βγ dimer are then able to activate further effectors until the α subunit acting as a GTPase mediates GTP hydrolysis (to GDP) resulting in its re-association with the βγ dimer. This then is the cycle of G-protein function.

SECOND MESSENGER SYSTEMS

Three major second messenger systems:

1 **Adenylyl cyclase/cAMP system**: the membrane glycoprotein adenylyl cyclase contains two cytoplasmic catalytic domains and 12 transmembrane regions. Stimulation by the G_s-α subunit activates adenylyl cyclase which converts ATP to cAMP (Mg^{2+}-dependent process). In some instances cAMP binds directly to ion channels; however, in most cases cAMP activates protein kinases. Protein kinase A (PKA) consists of two catalytic and two regulatory subunits. When two molecules of cAMP bind to the regulatory subunits the catalytic subunits are released and can phosphorylate proteins.
2 **Phosphoinositide system**: the membrane phospholipid phosphatidylinositol 4,5-bisphosphate (**PIP$_2$**) is subject to hydrolysis by two forms of phospholipase C (**PLC**) (one form is G-protein coupled the other is associated with neurotrophin-sensitive protein tyrosine kinase receptors). PIP_2 hydrolysis produces two second messengers, inositol triphosphate (**IP$_3$**) and diacylglycerol (**DAG**). The latter remains in the membrane and stimulates protein kinase C (**PKC**). IP_3 diffuses into the cytoplasm and binds to a specific endoplasmic reticulum (ER) receptor to release Ca^{2+}. Ca^{2+} then interacts with **calmodulin** (Ca^{2+}-binding protein) to form a complex (**CaM**) which modulates the activity of several proteins (some types of adenylyl cyclase, cytoskeletal proteins tau and MAP-2, and kinases, particularly CaM-dependent protein kinase II).
3 **Arachidonic acid (AA)/phospholipase A$_2$ system**: membrane phospholipids contain an unsaturated fatty acid arachidonic acid (AA) which can be released by the action of phospholipase A_2. AA can be metabolized to a variety of eicosanoids that act as messengers. AA is metabolized by the following:

Table 13.4

Lipoxygenase	$\Rightarrow$ **Leukotrienes**
Cyclooxygenase	$\Rightarrow$ **Prostaglandins** and thromboxanes
Cytochrome P-450	$\Rightarrow$ Epoxy-eicosatrienoic acid
Autooxidation	$\Rightarrow$ Hydroperoxy acid

ACETYLCHOLINE RECEPTORS

Some effects of ACh are mimicked by muscarine and others by nicotine. Muscarine and nicotine are both alkaloids (bitter tasting, nitrogen-containing substances usually derived from plants), and are found in amanita muscaria (fly agaric mushroom) and nicotania tabacum (tobacco plant) respectively. Hence muscarinic and nicotinic receptors.

Nicotinic receptors: ligand-gated ionotropic receptors with rapid responses (milliseconds) that are always excitatory. The membrane spanning pentameric neuronal nicotinic receptor contains a central cation-conducting pore of 0.65 nm diameter. It is made up of five glycoprotein subunits and two of these (designated α subunits) bind an ACh molecule each. Channel opening requires both α subunit sites be occupied, and this is facilitated by positive cooperativity. Intrinsic to this receptor is the ability to undergo desensitization.

Nicotinic receptors are found in striated muscles, postganglionic neurons (sympathetic and parasympathetic*) and chromaffin cells* of adrenal medulla. (*Also have muscarinic receptors.)

Muscarinic receptors: G-protein-coupled metabotropic receptors with slower responses that can be either excitatory or inhibitory. Five subtypes of muscarinic receptors M1–5. Muscarinic receptors are found in cardiac and smooth muscle with parasympathetic innervation, in sweat, salivary and tear glands. Agonists and antagonists at cholinergic receptors are shown in Table 13.6.

Table 13.5 Muscarinic receptor subtypes

Receptor subtype actions	M2 and M4	inhibit adenylyl cyclase (striatum)
	M1, M3 and M5	release inositol triphosphate (IP$_3$) and diacylglycerol (DAG)
		increase cAMP
		arachidonic acid metabolism
		(hindbrain; cerebellum)

Table 13.6 Cholinergic agonists and antagonists

Cholinergic agonists:	**carbachol** and **methacholine** (resistant tocholinesterase degradation and do not cross blood–brain barrier (BBB))
Nicotinic agonists:	**nicotine** and **methylcarbachol**
	succinylcholine and **decamethonium** (muscle receptor depolarization block, no central effects)
Nicotinic antagonists:	**hexamethonium** and **mecamylamine** (affinity for ganglia)
	+-tubocurarine and **gallamine** (affinity for muscle, no central effects)
Muscarinic agonists:	**muscarine** and **pilocarpine** and **arecoline**
Muscarinic antagonists:	**atropine** and **scopolamine**
	M1-**pirenzepine**

DOPAMINE RECEPTORS

G-protein-coupled and designated D_1–D_5. D_2 has two isoforms. Receptors fall into two groups: D_1-like (D_1 [subdivided further into D_{1A} and D_{1B}] and D_5) and D_2-like (D_2, D_3 and D_4). D_1-like linked via Gs to adenylate cyclase; D_2-like negatively coupled via G_i to adenylate cyclase.

D_1, D_2 and D_3 receptors are abundant in the nucleus accumbens, and olfactory tubercles. Additionally D_1 and D_2 also have a rich presence in the caudate and putamen ($D_2 > D_1$), and D_3 is predominant in limbic areas and the hypothalamus.

D_4 receptors have a high concentration in the frontal cortex, brainstem, and diencephalon while D_5 receptors are more localized to the hippocampus and hypothalamus.

Only D_2 and D_4 receptors have significant presence in the pituitary and the genes for these receptors are both carried on chromosome 11. D_2-like receptors (D_2, D_3, D_4) have both pre- and post-synaptic functions. As autoreceptors they can diminish cell firing and inhibit DA synthesis/release. D_1-like receptors have only post-synaptic functions.

Many DA receptor-binding drugs show little selectivity. However compounds with some selectivity are shown in Table 13.7:

Table 13.7

D_1 receptor agonists:	**SKF 38393**
D_2 receptor agonists:	**bromocriptine; apomorphine**
D_2 receptor antagonists:	**haloperidol: sulpiride; raclopride;**
	pimozide; spiperone; domperidone
D_3 receptor agonists:	**pergolide; quinpirole; 7-OH-DPAT**

ADRENOCEPTORS

G-protein-coupled receptors sensitive to noradrenaline and adrenaline.

Defined as α or β adrenoceptors on basis of agonist potency:

- *α adrenoceptor*: NA~Ad > isoprenaline (antagonized by phentolamine)
- *β adrenoceptor*: isoprenaline > Ad~NA (antagonized by propranolol).

Agonists/antagonists further distinguish:

- *α adrenoceptor*: α_1 and α_2
- *β adrenoceptor*: β_1, β_2 and β_3.

α_1 adrenoceptors are excitatory and post-synaptic. They are involved in smooth muscle contraction and glandular secretion.

α_2 adrenoceptors are inhibitory and both post- and pre-synaptic. Found in brain.

β_1 adrenoceptors are found mainly in heart tissue and within brain neurones.

β_2 adrenoceptors are more localized to glia and blood vessels.

SEROTONIN RECEPTORS

Four established classes of receptor: 5-HT_1, 5-HT_2, 5-HT_3 and 5-HT_4.

5-HT_1 receptors are further sub-divided into 5-HT_{1A}, 5-HT_{1B} and 5-HT_{1D} receptors and 5-HT_2 receptors are sub-divided into 5-HT_{2A}, 5-HT_{2B} and 5-HT_{2C} receptors. (NB 5-HT_{2C} receptor was previously called 5-HT_{1C}; hence no 5-HT_{1C} receptor.)

Serotonin receptors can be divided according to their second messenger systems:

- 5-HT_3 is an ionotropic ligand gated channel and is the exception
- 5-HT_{1A}, 5-HT_{1B}, 5-HT_{1D} and 5-HT_4 receptors are G-protein-linked to adenylate cyclase
- 5-HT_{2A}, 5-HT_{2B} and 5-HT_{2C} receptors are coupled to the phosphatidyl inositol system.

RECEPTOR ACTIONS: (ANIMAL AND HUMAN DATA)

- $5\text{-}HT_1$: receptors are inhibitory and negatively couple to cAMP.
- $5\text{-}HT_{1A}$: post-synaptic receptor (hippocampus and periaqueductal grey) – regulates impulsivity response to stress and resilience; pre-synaptic somatodendritic autoreceptor.
- $5\text{-}HT_{1B}$: functions as autoreceptor and possibly also as heteroreceptor on ACh, glutamate and dopamine neurones.
- $5\text{-}HT_{1D}$: functions as autoreceptor; inhibitory heteroreceptor function on trigeminal nerve terminal neuropeptide release.
- $5\text{-}HT_{2A}$: mediates increased capillary permeability, platelet aggregation, contraction of smooth muscle (blood vessels, gut, urinary tract and uterus). Located in basal ganglia, cortex and claustrum; mediate sensory perception – hallucinogenic effect of LSD.
- $5\text{-}HT_{2B}$: stimulation causes mild anxiety and hyperphagia (animal studies) and vasodilatation may be precipitant of migraine.
- $5\text{-}HT_{2C}$: possibly regulates CSF production. Other functions not yet clear but probably mediates anxiety and panic. Modify food intake.
- $5\text{-}HT_3$: wide distribution peripherally and centrally. Involved in cardiac, lung and intestinal activity, mediate vasodilatation, and stimulation causes pain, **nausea** and vomiting.
- $5\text{-}HT_4$: mediates cortisol secretion and contraction of colon and bladder. Centrally mediates striatal dopamine release.
- $5\text{-}HT_6$: implicated in attention, learning, memory.
- $5\text{-}HT_7$: implicated in depression and circadian rhythms.

Most serotonergic compounds act on several 5-HT receptor sub-types. Some (e.g. $5\text{-}HT_{1A}$ and $5\text{-}HT_{2C}$ anxiolytic and anxiogenic respectively) have opposing effects, and so the role of specific receptors is not yet fully known.

HISTAMINE RECEPTORS

Three subtypes: H_1, H_2 and H_3. H_1 and H_2 are coupled to G-proteins and act via phosphoinositide and adenylyl cyclase second messengers respectively.

- H_1 *receptors*: widely distributed both peripherally and centrally. Particularly dense in hypothalamus, cerebellum and limbic system. Selective agonist: 2-thiazolylethylamine. Antagonists: diphenhydramine and mepyramine. H_1 receptor activation stimulates wakefulness and suppresses slow-wave sleep.
- H_2 *receptors*: wide distribution in peripheral tissues and role in gastric acid secretion is of particular clinical importance. Centrally located in forebrain dopamine terminal areas such as striatum. Agonist: dimaprit. Antagonists: ranitidine and cimetidine.
- H_3 *receptor*: autoreceptor and heteroreceptor. Agonist: methylhistamine, Antagonist: thioperamide.

Clinically, H_1 receptor blockers cause sedation. Newer drugs (terfenadine, astemizole) do not cross BBB and therefore avoid this adverse effect.

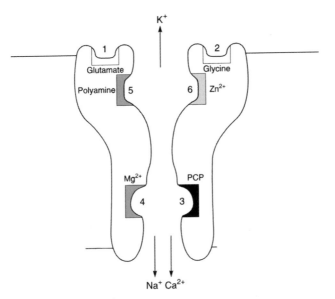

Figure 13.5 NMDA receptor complex

NMDA receptor complex:
1. L-glutamate binding site. Agonists promote high-conductance channel opening permitting Na^+ and Ca^{2+} entry.
2. Strychnine-insensitive glycine-binding site. Occupancy necessary for glutamate efficacy. Normal concentration saturates site and produces tonic stimulation.
3. Phencyclidine binding site (PCP). Also binds ketamine and dizocilpine (non-competitive antagonists). *Use-dependent blockade.*
4. Magnesium-binding site (Mg^{2+}). Voltage dependent. *Blockade.*
5. Polyamine binding site. Binds spermine and spermidine. *Facilitatory.*
6. Zinc binding site (Zn^{2+}). Voltage independent. *Blockade.*

EAA RECEPTORS (GLUTAMATE RECEPTORS) (see Figure 13.5)

Glutamate receptors are functionally heterogenous and can be ionotropic (ligand-gated channels) or metabotropic (G-protein coupled).

The ionotropic receptors are further characterized according to their prototypical agonist and named accordingly. Hence:

IONOTROPIC GLUTAMATE RECEPTORS

- AMPA (α-amino-3-hydroxy-5-methyl-4-isoxazole propionic acid)
- NMDA (N-methyl-D-aspartate)
- kainite/kainic acid (extracted from seaweed).

Agonists with some selectivity: quisqualate (AMPA); ibotenic acid (NMDA); domoic acid (kainite).

All three ionotropic receptor channels are permeable to Na^+ and K^+ but only NMDA receptors are additionally permeable to Ca^{2+}.

AMPA and kainite receptors are central to fast excitatory transmission and give rise to fast EPSPs.

NMDA receptor EPSPs are slow and involve Ca^{2+} activation of calcium-dependent processes.

AMPA and NMDA receptors interact such that the NMDA receptor channel is sensitive to voltage-dependent blockade by Mg^{2+} ions (Magnesium ion-binding site). This block can be removed by depolarization brought about by AMPA receptor activation. NMDA receptors also have an important interaction with glycine. Glycine binds to a separate site on the NMDA receptor complex (NMDA-rc) and its occupancy of this site is essential for activation of the receptor by glutamate. (NB the NMDA receptor complex glycine-binding site is not sensitive to strychnine but is sensitive to the agonist D-serine.) The NMDA-rc also has other regulatory sites:

- *PCP (phencyclidine) site*: binds ketamine and dizocilpine (MK801). These non-competitive antagonists exhibit use-dependent blockade of the channel
- *polyamine site*: binds spermidine and spermine (involved in tissue growth). Facilitates NMDA-rc transmission (can both $\uparrow$ and $\downarrow$)
- *zinc ion (Zn^{2+})-binding site*: voltage-independent block of NMDA-rc.

METABOTROPIC GLUTAMATE RECEPTORS

Seven receptors (mGluR1–7) grouped according to second messenger coupling, pharmacology and aa sequence homology: (trans-ACPD is a rigid glutamate analogue that has selective agonist activity at metabotropic glutamate receptors).

- *group 1*: mGluR1 and mGluR5 use phosphoinositide system and are sensitive to quisqualate and trans-ACPD
- *group 2*: mGluR2 and mGluR3 inhibit adenylate cyclase and are sensitive only to trans-ACPD not to quisqualate
- *group 3*: mG1uR4, mG1uR6 and mG1uR7 inhibit adenylate cyclase and are insensitive to both trans-ACPD and quisqualate. Group 3 receptors are instead sensitive to phosphorylated aas and possibly function aas autoreceptors inhibiting glutamate release.

Continuous neuronal stimulation by EAAs can lead to cell damage and death. This is called **excitotoxicity** and is possibly the basis of injury in epilepsy, ischaemia, amyotrophic lateral sclerosis and Huntingdon's disease.

Glutamate receptors are involved in the phenomenon of long-term potentiation (LTP), thought to be the basis of learning and memory storage.

GABA RECEPTORS (see Figure 13.6)

Three GABA receptors: $GABA_A$, $GABA_B$, $GABA_C$.

- *$GABA_A$*: ionotropic receptor (ligand-gated channel) mediating fast post-synaptic IPSPs and permeable to Cl^- ions. Can be blocked by competitive (bicuculline – binds to GABA-binding site) and non-competitive (picrotoxin) antagonists producing

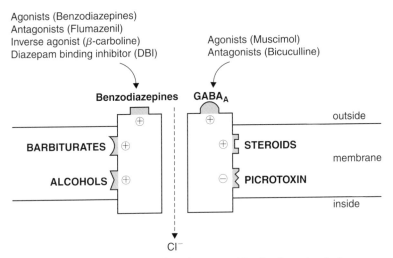

Agonists (Benzodiazepines)
Antagonists (Flumazenil)
Inverse agonist (β-carboline)
Diazepam binding inhibitor (DBI)

Agonists (Muscimol)
Antagonists (Bicuculline)

GABA$_A$ receptor complex consists of two α and β subunits and a single
γ subunit. Pentameric structure forms intrinsic chloride (Cl$^-$) channel
that is positively and negatively modulated by a variety of ligands and drugs

Figure 13.6 GABA$_A$ receptor complex

convulsions. Benzodiazepines, barbiturates, ethanol and anaesthetic steroids potentiate the effects of GABA on GABA$_A$ receptors. The GABA$_A$ receptor consists of five glycoprotein subunits and has a variety of modulatory sites. Specificity for subunits – of newer hypnotics such as **zopiclone** – diminishes adverse effects (dependence, memory loss). Action of benzodiaepines can be blocked by antagonists such as **flumazenil**.

- *GABA$_B$*: G-protein-coupled receptors that are pre- and post-synaptic. GABA$_B$ receptor G-proteins interact directly with ion channels (activate K$^+$ channels and inhibit Ca^{2+} channels), activate phospholipase A$_2$, or inhibit adenylate cyclase. Selective agonist: baclofen and saclofen. Antagonists: 2-hydroxysaclofen and phaclofen.
- *GABA$_C$*: like GABA$_A$ receptors, form Cl$^-$ channels but consist of novel subunits ρ1 and ρ2 (found in retina). Insensitive to bicuculline and baclofen and not affected by barbiturates or benzodiazepines.

GABA plays a crucial regulatory role and inhibits neurotransmission through both pre- and post-synaptic mechanisms. GABA$_B$ receptors implicated in amine release, cognition and absence seizures.

GLYCINE RECEPTORS

The glycine receptor is an ionotropic receptor containing a ligand-gated channel for Cl$^-$ ions which produces fast post-synaptic IPSPs. The receptor is a pentamer composed of two subunits ($3\alpha, 2\beta$). **Strychnine**, derived from the seeds of a tree (*Strychnos nux vomica*), is a potent glycine receptor antagonist. It binds to the α subunit of the receptor causing muscle stiffness, convulsions and death.

Psychopharmacology

14

The mechanisms by which most psychotropics (including antipsychotics, antidepressants and mood stabilizers) alleviate psychiatric symptoms are not fully understood. Lists of drug interactions, cautions/contraindications in liver or renal impairment and issues of drug safety in pregnancy/breast-feeding can be found in the appendices of the *British National Formulary*.

Rare psychiatric associations of certain drugs include: depression (methyldopa, digoxin, clonidine, propranolol, oral contraceptive pill, cimetidine); psychosis (steroids, chloroquine, vigabatrin, benzodiazepines (BZDs)). Many of these associations overlap.

ANTIPSYCHOTICS (FORMERLY NEUROLEPTICS/MAJOR TRANQUILLIZERS)

It is thought that all antipsychotics must exhibit some degree of D_2 blockade in order to be effective. However, despite wide variations in D_2 blockade (i.e. **potency**), no antipsychotic (with the exception of clozapine, which actually exhibits relatively low D_2 affinity) has proven to be more efficacious than any other in the treatment of positive psychotic symptoms.

Potency is thus not a measure of clinical effectiveness (e.g. clozapine is a low-potency drug). The choice of drug in individual cases is instead determined largely by cost/availability, side-effect profile (desirable as well as undesirable), the patient's history/wishes and the prescriber's experience.

With any antipsychotic the clinical effect is generally not seen for at least the first week of treatment, though side-effects (such as sedation) may appear much sooner. Switching antipsychotics is best achieved by careful cross-titration, and though there is no clear dependence syndrome there may be cholinergic rebound if treatment is stopped suddenly.

Receptor interactions: three major dopamine-mediated pathways:

- *Nigrostriatal* (motor): substantia nigra pars compacta (A9) → striatum. D_2 receptor blockade causes EPS (percentages are for typicals) – parkinsonism (20 per cent), akathisia (20–25 per cent) [a pervasive sense of restlessness and an important cause of suicide], tardive dyskinesia (5 per cent) (↑ risk with prolonged use, high dose, elderly, female; absent during sleep), dystonic reactions (10 per cent). Dystonic reactions tend to be subjectively painful before they are clinically obvious.

- *Mesolimbic* [ventral tegmental area (VTA) A10 $\rightarrow$ limbic system (amygdala, nucleus accumbens, pyriform cortex, lateral septal nucleus)] and *mesocortical* [VTA $\rightarrow$ septo-hippocampal region and frontal cortex]: perception, thinking, emotion. Post-synaptic D_2 receptor blockade responsible for clinical antipsychotic effect; $\uparrow$ VTA selectivity = $\downarrow$ EPS.
- *Tuberoinfundibular* (hormonal): hypothalamic arcuate nucleus (A12) $\rightarrow$ median eminence. Dopamine acts on anterior pituitary lobe mammotroph D_2 receptors to suppress prolactin-release-inhibiting factor. Antagonism causes hyperprolacti-naemia and sexual side-effects: galactorrhoea, gynaecomastia, amenorrhoea, impotence, infertility, breast cancer, osteoporosis.

Effect on other receptors:

- *adrenergic* (α_1) blockade: dose-dependent postural hypotension (particularly with phenothiazines in the elderly), necessitating careful titration when starting antipsy-chotics with high α_1 affinity (e.g. clozapine, risperidone, most typicals). Additional effects are dizziness, tachycardia and ejaculatory failure/impotence (an important cause of non-adherence with psychotropic medication).
- *anticholinergic*: central – seizures, pyrexia and possible $\downarrow$ cognitive functioning; peripheral – blurred vision, urinary retention, constipation (especially clozapine), sinus tachycardia, amnesia and reduced secretions (dry mouth). Use with caution in glaucoma and prostatism.
- *histaminergic* (H_1) blockade: sedation, weight gain and possibly anti-emetic effect via action on chemosensitive trigger zone.
- *serotonergic* (5-HT) blockade: sexual disturbance (5-HT_{2A}) and weight gain (5-HT_{2C}). Also believed to be important in atypicals' mechanism of action.

Effect on other systems:

- *endocrine* system: $\uparrow$ prolactin and melanocyte stimulating hormone (MSH). $\downarrow$ antidiuretic hormone (ADH), adrenocorticotrophic hormone (ACTH) and possibly growth hormone (GH).
- *cardiovascular*: QTc (i.e. corrected for heart rate) prolongation (>450 ms) may lead to the potentially fatal ventricular arrhythmia torsade de pointes. Link more clearly established with typicals than atypicals (particularly pimozide and thioridazine), but sertindole and ziprasidone also implicated. Main hazards are high dose/mult-iple antipsychotics and pre-existing risk factors (e.g. female, elderly, electrolyte disturbance, long QT-syndrome, cardiac history). In these circumstances electro-cardiogram (ECG) monitoring is advised.
- *autonomic*: blood pressure and temperature regulation (dose dependent).
- *skin*: photosensitivity and allergic dermatitis (urticarial, oedematous, petechial and maculopapular). Occur early in treatment and more so with low-potency drugs. Chlorpromazine in particular can discolour the skin, especially upon exposure to the sun (necessitating sun-screen etc. as appropriate).
- *haematological*: leucopaenia, agranulocytosis (incidence of 1:500 000, more likely with chlorpromazine and thioridazine), thrombocytopaenia, haemolytic anaemia and leucocytosis.
- *jaundice*: 1:1000. Strongly associated with phenothiazines (especially chlorpro-mazine and thioridazine), which cause a 'chemical' obstructive jaundice that may be part of a photosensitivity reaction.

- $\downarrow$ *seizure threshold*: dose-dependent, $\uparrow$ risk the more sedative the drug. Estimated 10-fold increase in seizures in non-epileptics receiving antipsychotic or antidepressant medication. Clozapine most epileptogenic. Also recommended to avoid chlorpromazine, loxapine and depots (due to pharmacokinetics) in epilepsy.
- *eyes*: irreversible pigmentation of retina (similar to retinitis pigmentosa) seen with phenothiazines (especially thioridazine), which can lead to blindness even after treatment cessation. Deposits in lens and cornea, not associated with change in visual acuity. Discoloration of conjunctiva.

Other side-effects:

- *emotional blunting*: although this may be desirable in highly aroused individuals, it can be difficult to distinguish between apathy caused by the disease and that caused by the medication.
- *fluid regulation*: up to 1/5 may drink excessively. NB: Excessive smoking can reduce urine concentration.
- *aggression*: aside from possible paradoxical reactions, side-effects such as akathisia may cause a medicated individual to be more irritable and impulsive.

Interactions:

- *Sedation*: sedative antipsychotics likely to potentiate sedative action of other drugs (e.g. opioid analgesics, antihistamines, alcohol, barbiturates and benzodiazepines).
- *EPS*: $\uparrow$ risk with contraceptive pill, opioid analgesics and psychotropic polypharmacy.

TARDIVE DYSKINESIA (TD)

Affects 45–50 per cent of patients (men and women equally) treated long term (months to years) with antipsychotics. Risk/incidence is greatest early in treatment but increases with age and can occur in elderly independent of antipsychotic exposure. Risk of TD is not dose related and is not associated with the use of anticholinergic medication.

Exact aetiology is unknown but the responsible antipsychotic and any concomitant anticholinergic medication should be gradually reduced/withdrawn.

Subsequent management may include clozapine, benzodiazepines, tetrabenzine, neurosurgery (pallidotomy).

NEUROLEPTIC MALIGNANT SYNDROME (NMS)

An idiosynchratic reaction (incidence up to 1 per cent) to certain psychotropics that carries a fatality rate of up to 10 per cent. Most commonly associated with antipsychotics (typicals > atypicals), but has been reported with antidepressants and mood stabilizers.

Can occur at any stage of treatment but $\uparrow$ risk within first 7 days (28 with depot), high starting dose/rapid upward titration, psychotropic polypharmacy (including drugs of different classes) and concurrent systemic disease. Evolves rapidly over 3 days, lasting up to 2 weeks if untreated.

Diagnosed if all three of the following present (in someone taking a relevant medication):

- *hyperthermia** (>38°C): 're-setting' of homeostatic control + ↑ heat production secondary to muscle activity
- *marked extrapyramidal effects*: at least two of muscular rigidity*, cogwheeling, oculogyric crisis, trismus, opisthotonus, sialorrhoea, retrocollis, choreoathetoid movements, tremulousness* or dysphagia
- *Autonomic dysfunction*: at least two of tachycardia*, hypertension (↑ diastolic >20 mmHg) or lability of blood pressure, urinary incontinence or marked diaphoresis*

OR two of the above and at least one of the following:

- fluctuating consciousness*
- serum creatinine kinase >1000 IU/ml
- leucocytosis.

Other signs include abnormal liver function tests (LFTs), hyperkalaemia, rhabdomyolisis (myoglobinaemia may lead to renal damage), diffuse slowing on EEG*, dehydration* and proteinuria*.
(* seen in >90 per cent of cases).

Management: the syndrome is a serious medical emergency and the antipsychotic must be stopped immediately.

- Bromocriptine (DA agonist) can be used to reverse anti-dopaminergic effects.
- Dantroline can be used to relieve muscle spasm.
- If antipsychotic medication is deemed necessary post-recovery, there should be at least a 2-week interval and a structurally different antipsychotic should be used.

TYPICALS

Typicals have a narrow therapeutic index for extra-pyramidal side-effects (EPS).
Tend to attain similar levels of D_2 receptor binding in the striatum and cortex.

- *Phenothiazines*: highly sedative (antihistamine and α-adrenergic action)
  - *aliphatic side-chain*: chlorpromazine and promazine (the most sedating phenothiazines), methotrimeprazine/levomepromazine
  - *piperazine side-chain*: fluphenazine (depot) and trifluoperazine (least sedating but ↑ EPS; also used as an anxiolytic and antiemetic), perphenazine, prochlorperazine
  - *piperidine side-chain*: thioridazine (restricted licence in UK), pipothiazine (depot), pericyazine (some success in controlling aggressive behaviour).
- *Thioxanthenes*: flupenthixol (mostly used in depot form; has antidepressant action), zuclopenthixol (depot).
- *Butyrophenones*: haloperidol, droperidol (withdrawn in UK), benperidol. Little/ no anticholinergic action and so ↑ risk of EPS over phenothiazines.
- *Diphenylbutylpiperidines*: pimozide (fewer side-effects as relatively specific for dopamine receptors, but significant association with cardiac-mediated sudden death), fluspirilene (no longer prescribed).
- *Substituted benzamide*: sulpiride.

HALOPERIDOL

Discovered by Janssen. Non-linear dose–response curve, with ↑ EPS at higher doses. Peak plasma level within 6 h of oral and 20 min of i.m. administration (i.m. dose equivalent to double oral dose). Half-life approx. 20 h. Excreted in breast-milk.

Possible interactions: inhibits metabolism of tricyclics (can lead to TCA toxicity); prolonged concurrent carabamazepine use may ↓ plasma haloperidol level.

CHLORPROMAZINE

Discovered by Charpentier, who was trying to create an antihistamine for anaesthetic use. Antipsychotic efficacy established in early 1950s (Delay and Deniker).

Sedative. >90 per cent protein bound (albumin). Onset of sedative action within 60 min of oral and 30 min of i.m. administration (postural hypotension common, lasting up to 2 h). Marked first-pass metabolism; higher plasma levels achieved by i.m. route. Half-life approx 30 h. Excreted in breast-milk. Induces its own hepatic metabolism. ↑ δ and θ-wave and ↓ fast β-wave activity on EEG.

Possible interactions: additive effect with antihistamines in prolonging QTc; TCAs may ↑ chlorpromazine plasma level; ↑ plasma lithium levels (risk of lithium encephalopathy), while lithium and orphenadrine may significantly ↓ chlorpromazine plasma level.

ATYPICALS

Atypicals have a wide therapeutic index for EPS.

Tend to attain higher D_2 receptor binding in the cortex than the striatum. Less overall D_2 occupancy than typicals but greater interaction with D_1, D_4, 5-HT_{2C} and 5-HT_3 receptors. They also antagonize 5-HT_{2A} to varying degrees, which is thought to further decrease their propensity for EPS and implicates serotonin (which plays a regulatory role in striatal dopaminergic transmission) in their mechanism of action.

- Clozapine (dibenzodiazepine)
- Risperidone (benzisoxazole)
- Amisulpiride (substituted benzamide) [treats negative symptoms of schizophrenia at low doses and positive symptoms at higher doses]
- Olanzapine (thienobenzodiazepine)
- Sertindole (imidazolidinone) [never made it to US market and restricted in UK due to association with arrhythmias and sudden death]
- Quetiapine (dibenzothiazepine)
- Zotepine (substituted dibenzothiazepine tricyclic)
- Aripiprazole (quinolinone derivative)
- Ziprasidone (benzothiazolylpiperazine).

Current evidence suggests atypicals are superior to placebo in symptom reduction, and less likely to induce movement disorders than typicals. However, the vast majority of clinical trials on atypicals are relatively short and provide little information on long-term outcome. Although no more efficacious than typicals, they may be more effective since they are generally better tolerated.

CLOZAPINE

The first atypical. Trialled in 1960s, later withdrawn due to incidences of NMS and agranulocytosis. Reintroduced when shown to be more effective than other antipsychotics in treatment-resistant schizophrenia. Also thought to have extremely low potential for extrapyramidal side-effects (has been used as a treatment for tardive dyskinesia) and to be of similar effectiveness to amisulpiride in treating negative symptoms. Does not ↑ serum prolactin.

Peak plasma levels in 1–4 hours, half-life 16 hours, target plasma range 350 to 600 μg/l. Active metabolite norclozapine.

The patient, prescribing doctor and dispensing pharmacy must all be registered with the Clozapine Patient Monitoring Service (CPMS), which regulates the administration of clozapine according to strict haematological protocols. Any patient suspected of having an infection (pyrexia, sore throat, rhinorrhoea etc.) should have an immediate infection screen and white cell count performed.

Side-effects:

- *sedation and postural hypotension*: can be marked, necessitates slow initial titration; ↑ risk if used with quetiapine or chloropromazine
- *reversible neutropenia*: 3 per cent, ↑ risk if used with phenothiazines or flupenthixol
- *agranulocytosis*: 0.8 per cent, possible ↑ risk if used with risperidone; potentially fatal
- *sialorrhoea*: common
- *seizures*: 3–5 per cent, ↑ risk if used with chlorpromazine, loxapine or zotepine
- *glucose intolerance and weight gain*: baseline measurement with subsequent monitoring recommended
- *myocarditis and cardiomyopathy*: especially first 3 months; potentially fatal
- *pyrexia*: may complicate diagnosis of infection
- *jaundice*.

All selective serotonin re-uptake inhibitors (SSRIs) (except citalopram) ↑ plasma clozapine levels; phenytoin ↓ plasma levels. Clozapine potentiates effects of warfarin and digoxin, and the sedative action of alcohol.

RISPERIDONE

Although licensed up to 16 mg/day, risperidone is generally not prescribed above 8 mg/day (2–6 mg said to be optimal) due to occurrence of EPS. Also associated with significant hyperprolactineamia.

Available in depot form as a suspension (therefore no flexibility of dosing) which must be given every two weeks (no flexibility of timing). Anecdotally, may have a lower therapeutic index for EPS than oral risperidone.

Other side-effects: *RISPERIDONE*

Rashes
Insomnia
Sedation
Priapism
Emesis
Retrograde ejaculation

*I*ncontinence
*D*yspepsia
*O*cular disturbances
*N*eutropenia but not agranulocytosis
*E*nzyme abnormalities (liver).

OLANZAPINE

Biochemically similar to clozapine, weight gain ($\uparrow$ risk if used with lithium or valproate) and glucose intolerance are of major concern in some patients. Again, baseline measurement and monitoring are advisable. However, olanzapine is generally well tolerated (though initial sedation can be a problem); manufacturer states that a therapeutic dose can be started directly (10 mg) without any need for titration.

Thought to have antidepressant properties, and also licensed for use in acute mania. Metabolism (cytochrome p450 1A2) induced by smoking; heavy smoking may reduce olanzapine's (and other psychotropics' such as TCAs and clozapine) effectiveness; conversely, fluvoxamine inhibits this isoenzyme and so may $\uparrow$ olanzapine level. Carbamazepine can $\downarrow$ olanzapine half-life by up to 20 per cent through hepatic induction.

Available in 'velotab' form for rapid ingestion, but patient must still swallow the dissolved tablet in order to receive the drug (i.e. it is not absorbed via the buccal mucosa).

Other side-effects: $\uparrow$ in *OLANZP*

*O*edema
*L*iver enzymes
*A*ppetite $\uparrow$
*N*eutropenia
*Z*edation (usually transient)
*P*rolactinaemia (transient).

QUETIAPINE

Like olanzapine, has a chemical structure related to clozapine. However, pharmacologically very different with predominant action on D_2, 5-HT_{2A} and H_1 receptors. Effective against positive and negative symptoms of schizophrenia and has emerging role in the treatment of bipolar disorder.

Is very atypical with little or no EPS or hyperprolactinaemia, but can cause weight gain via action on histamine receptors. Typical side-effects include sedation, dry mouth, constipation and dizziness. Associated with liver and thyroid function test changes.

ARIPIPRAZOLE

Marketed as a new class of antipsychotic – a partial dopamine (D_2) agonist. Thought to 'stabilize' dopamine function by enhancing neurotransmission in deficient areas and attenuate dopamine transmission in areas of overactivity.

Good side-effect profile with a theoretically lower incidence of EPS. However, significant association with akathisia, which is believed to be mediated through its action at 5-HT_{1A} (partial agonist) and 5-HT_{2A} (high-affinity antagonist) receptors. Severity of akathisia between that of typicals and other atypicals. Has no anticholinergic effects, does not cause hyperprolactinaemia and is a low-affinity antagonist at α_1 and H_1 receptors.

Ketoconazole, erythromicin, quinidine and fluoxetine raise plasma aripiprazole levels. Carbamazepine $\downarrow$ plasma levels.

ZOTEPINE

High affinity for D_1 and D_2. Increases dopaminergic activity at low doses, inhibitory at high doses (hence dose-dependent effect on prolactin levels). Also acts at 5-HT$_{2A}$, 5-HT$_{2C}$, 5-HT$_6$ and 5-HT$_7$ receptors. Some benefit against negative symptoms, thought to be mediated via its serotonergic activity and (additional) noradrenaline (NA) re-uptake inhibition.

Metabolized primarily by N-demethylation to norzotepine, which also has an affinity for dopaminergic receptors. BZDs increase plasma level.

Significant association with weight gain and QTc prolongation. Also associated with drowsiness, akathisia, abnormal LFTs and anticholinergic side-effects.

ZIPRASIDONE

Used in USA and in some EU countries (not UK). Higher 5-HT$_{2A}$: D_2 affinity ratio than most other antipsychotics. Has no anticholinergic effect and is less sedative than clozapine and olanzapine, with low potential for hypotension (useful in elderly).

Possible anxiolytic and antidepressant properties (perhaps because of weak serotonin/noradrenaline reuptake inhibition).

Typical side-effects are headache, nausea and vomiting, insomnia, tremor. Very little weight gain/anticholinergic effect. Available in i.m. form.

AMISULPIRIDE

Relatively specific for D_2 with virtually no activity at non-DA receptors. Said to be effective against primary $-$ve symptoms at low doses (by antagonizing presynaptic DA receptors and so $\uparrow$ DA activity), and against $+$ve symptoms at higher doses (by antagonizing postsynaptic DA receptors).

Associated with prolactinaemia and EPS at higher doses. Minimally metabolized, excreted largely unchanged in the urine. May be used as an adjunct to clozapine in treatment-resistant schizophrenia.

ANTIPSYCHOTIC DEPOT INJECTIONS

Depots tend to be associated with higher incidences of EPS and other side-effects than their oral equivalents. Frequency of administration can be adjusted to help establish optimum cost/benefit ratio for individual patients. Generally, *f*lupent(h)ixol and *f*luphenazine decanoate can be administered relatively *f*requently (every 2 weeks), whereas haloperidol decanoate and pipothiazine palmitate are usually administered 4-weekly.

Zuclopenthixol can be administered in two forms:

- zu*clop*enthixol *ac*etate (*Clop*ixol-*Ac*uphase): *ac*ute illnesses (onset 2 hours, lasts up to 72 hours).
- zuclopenthixol *dec*anoate (every 2 weeks): *dep*ot treatment.

The risperidone depot Risperdal must be administered every 2 weeks as it has a much narrower pharmacokinetic profile than other depots. Risperidone is not actually released into the system until just over 2 weeks post-injection, and peaks at 3 weeks post-injection. Hence there is likely to be a delay of about one month (time lag for release + time lag for clinical effect) on initially starting the depot, and changes in dose will not alter the drug level for 3 weeks.

MANAGEMENT OF SIDE-EFFECTS

Establish cause – is problem due to medication? → Is medication necessary? → Minimize effective dose → Consider alternatives (e.g. typical to atypical, depot to oral) → Consult colleagues/see Maudsley Prescribing Guidelines for advice on specific side-effect problems.

Approximate doses of oral antipsychotics (mg) equivalent to chlorpromazine 100 mg (NB in the order displayed, for many, the dose doubles):

*R*ich *P*rivate *H*ospital *Tr*usts *L*ove *C*heap *Th*erapeutic *S*ervices

*R*isperidone	0.75
*P*imozide	1.5
*H*aloperidol	2.5
*Tr*ifluoperazine	5.0
*L*oxapine	10–20
*C*lozapine	50
*Th*ioridazine	100
*S*ulpiride	200 (amisulpride 100).

It is recommended that no patient receive more than a total combined equivalent of 2000 mg chlorpromazine over 24 hours. However, this must not extrapolate beyond any individual drug's maximum daily dosage.

General advice would be to use antipsychotics with caution in patients on sedatives, the elderly (↑ risk of orthostatic hypotension), those with cardiac/liver disease or movement disorders and blood dyscrasias. Warn about sedation. If antipsychotics must be given in pregnancy, typicals preferred as greater evidence base (i.e. have been used for longer).

Overdose: marked EPS, hypotension, sedation. Possible cardiac/autonomic instability.

ANTIDEPRESSANTS

Chance discovery in 1950s. Imipramine (TCA) had been developed as a chlorpromazine analogue and iproniazid (MAOI) was developed for the treatment of tuberculosis.

The **monoamine hypothesis** of depression proposed a functional deficiency of catecholamines (NA, DA) and indoleamines (5-HT) and served as a useful model for the development of antidepressants and understanding their actions.

Antidepressants classes have arisen on the basis of chemical structure and principal action. Most antidepressants act on serotonin, noradrenaline and dopamine neurotransmission.

TRICYCLIC ANTIDEPRESSANTS (TCAs) OR MONOAMINE RE-UPTAKE INHIBITORS (MARIs)

Tricyclics have a three-ring structure. The number of methyl groups attached to the side-chain nitrogen determines whether a TCA is tertiary (two groups) or secondary (one group) amine. TCAs block the re-uptake of noradrenaline and serotonin (2° amines > effect on NA re-uptake; 3° amines > effect on serotonin re-uptake). This is thought to be the basis of their therapeutic effect.

Effects on other receptors lead to their side-effects:

- *muscarine receptors*: dry mouth, blurred vision, urinary retention, constipation (less severe with 2° TCAs)
- *histamine receptors*: sedation and weight gain
- *adrenoceptors*: postural hypotension, sexual dysfunction
- membrane **stab**ilization (sodium channel blockade); cardiotoxic effects (**s**yncope, **t**achycardia, **a**rrhythmias, **b**lood pressure drop) and reduction of seizure threshold. ECG shows flattened T waves, prolongation of QT interval and depression of ST segment.

Generally 3° amine TCAs are more potent and more sedating.
Notes on individual antidepressants:

- *Amitriptyline*: has mild analgesic properties. Can be administered intramuscularly (i.m.) and intravenously (i.v.).
- *Amoxapine*: related to antipsychotic loxapine and can cause tardive dyskinesia.
- *Clomipramine*: noted for serotonergic effect; and is indicated for use in phobic and obsessional states in addition to depression. Can be given i.m. or i.v.
- *Dothiepin*: a derivative of amitriptyline, has fewer autonomic adverse effects and is somewhat less cardiotoxic. Sedative.
- *Doxepin*: a derivative of amitriptyline; because of serotonergic interaction has anxio-lytic properties.
- *Imipramine*: is additionally used for nocturnal enuresis in children.
- *Lofepramine*: fewer anticholinergic and cardiotoxic effects. It is less sedating and safer in overdose than most other TCAs.
- *Maprotiline*: is a tetracyclic compound; it lowers the seizure threshold.
- *Mianserin*: is a tetracyclic compound; it shows minimal cardiotoxicity and has few anticholinergic effects. Its main adverse effect is sedation.
- *Nortriptyline*: like imipramine, can be used for nocturnal enuresis in children.
- *Protriptyline*: has very little sedative effect.
- *Trimipramine*: has very strong sedative effect.

SELECTIVE SEROTONIN RE-UPTAKE INHIBITORS (SSRIs)

Defined by principal action on serotonin re-uptake inhibition; however, structurally distinct and have a number of effects on a variety of neurotransmitters. Used widely as first-line antidepressants because of better tolerability and safety than TCAs.

SSRIs: **fluoxetine, fluvoxamine, sertraline, paroxetine** and **citalopram**. S-enantiomer of citalopram (escitalopram) marketed as separate antidepressant. All are indicated for use in depressive illness and some have additional indications:

$$
\left.
\begin{array}{l}
\text{\emph{F}luoxetine} \\
\text{\emph{F}luvoxamine} \\
\text{\emph{P}aroxetine} \\
\text{Citalo\emph{p}ram}
\end{array}
\right\}
\begin{array}{l}
\left.
\begin{array}{l}
\text{Bulimia nervosa} \\
\text{(\emph{F}ood disorder)}
\end{array}
\right\} \\
\left.
\begin{array}{l}
\text{} \\
\text{\emph{P}anic disorder}
\end{array}
\right.
\end{array}
\left.
\begin{array}{l}
\\
\\
\end{array}
\right\}
\text{OCD}
$$

Approximate half-lives of SSRIs: 1 day: fluvoxamine, paroxetine and sertraline*
2 days: citalopram/escitalopram
3 days: fluoxetine*

*Fluoxetine and sertraline have active metabolites with much longer half-lives.

Drugs with short half-lives can precipitate withdrawal effects – especially paroxetine.

Low concentrations of SSRIs (in particular fluoxetine) appear in breast-milk.

Most adverse effects are experienced at the beginning of treatment and gradually diminish. All the SSRIs except citalopram (and escitalopram) inhibit cytochrome P450 enzymes. Paroxetine and fluoxetine inhibit P450-2D6 and interact with opiates, TCAs and antipsychotics. Fluvoxamine inhibits P450-1A2 and interacts with theophylline, caffeine and clozapine.

Fluoxetine: *FLUOXETINE*

*F*ever
*L*iver function tests abnormalities
*U*rticarial and other allergic reactions
*O*rgasmic dysfunction (delay)
e*X*tra-pyramidal side-effects
*E*cchymoses
*T*ension
*I*nsomnia
*N*ausea
*E*mesis.

(NB with *approximate* increasing frequency: last four are most frequent: tension/anxiety, insomnia, nausea and vomiting.)

Paroxetine and ***fluvoxamine***: common adverse effects – nausea and vomiting, headaches, dry mouth and sedation. Paroxetine does not lower seizure threshold but does have a withdrawal syndrome. It also ↑ plasma levels of olanzapine, risperidone and TCAs.

SSRI *DIS*CONTINUATION SYNDROME

DIScontinuation: **D**isequilibrium e.g. **D**izziness, **I**ncreased dreams and **I**nsomnia, **S**ensory abnormalities e.g. electric **S**hock sensation. Also get mood changes, somatic and gastrointestinal symptoms.

MONOAMINE OXIDASE INHIBITORS (MAOIs)

Most MAOIs (**phenelzine, isocarboxacid** and **tranylcypromine**) irreversibly inhibit *both* monoamine oxidases A and B. **Moclobemide** is a *selective* MAOI that exerts reversible inhibition of MAO-A. Moclo*B*emide is only MAOI to contain the letter '*B*' yet is the only one that does *not* act on MAO-B.

Normally, orally ingested tyramine undergoes MAO metabolism in the intestinal mucosa and the liver. MAO inhibition allows **tyramine** to enter the circulation and results in the prolonged release of noradrenaline. (NA is released by tyramine from neurones and its subsequent degradation is slowed because of MAO inhibition.) This results in sweating, headache, nausea and vomiting and a marked rise in blood pressure which can cause cerebral bleeding. It is commonly referred to as the 'cheese reaction' because cheese is particularly rich in tyramine and its ingestion produces marked adverse effects. Substances and foods that need to be avoided when consuming MAOIs are:

ABCDEFG

*A*lcohol – chianti, red wines and beer
*B*road bean pods
*C*heeses (exceptions – *C*ream and *C*ottage cheeses)
*D*rugs*
*E*xtracts of meat and yeast (Marmite, Bovril)
*F*ish, especially smoked or pickled (fresh fish is relatively safe)
*G*ame.

* drugs: direct and indirectly acting sympathomimetics (amphetamine, phenyl-propanolamine). NB can often be found in nasal decongestants and cough mixtures.

ABCDEFGHI

*A*ntidepressants (tricyclics)
*B*arbiturates
*C*ocaine, pethidine and other narcotics
L-*D*opa
*E*phedrine
*F*enfluramine
*G*eneral anaesthetics
anti*H*ypertensives
*I*nsulin.

In addition to the many possible drug and food interactions, MAOIs have several adverse effects related to receptor/metabolic actions:

- muscarinic action causing dry mouth, sweating, blurred vision, urinary hesitancy and constipation
- sympatheticomimetic action (dose related) causing weight gain, hypertension, restlessness
- serotonergic action causing **serotonin syndrome** with SSRIs or L-tryptophan
- postural hypotension and ankle oedema
- agitation, nervousness and tremor

- paraesthesiae (hands/feet) and peripheral neuropathy because of pyridoxine deficiency
- increased appetite and weight gain
- sleep disturbance and sexual dysfunction
- jaundice and hepatocellular necrosis.

ATYPICAL AND NOVEL ANTIDEPRESSANTS

- *Duloxetine*: dual action antidepressant blocking re-uptake of both noradrenaline and serotonin.
- *Flupenthixol*: thioxanthene that has antidepressant properties at low dose.
- *Mirtazapine*: dual action antidepressant which enhances serotonergic and noradrenergic neurotransmission. Also known as noradrenaline and serotonin-specific antidepressant (NaSSa). Antagonist at $5\text{-}HT_2$, $5\text{-}HT_3$, H_1 and pre-synaptic α_2 receptors.
- *Nefazodone*: $5\text{-}HT_2$ and α_1 receptor antagonist which also inhibits both serotonin and noradrenaline uptake. Inhibits CYP 3A: $\uparrow$ plasma levels of carbamazepine, atypicals and antihistamines.
- *Reboxetine*: selective noradrenaline re-uptake inhibitor. α_2 adrenoceptor antagonist.
- *Trazodone*: histaminergic and α_1 adrenoceptor antagonist. It is a serotonin re-uptake inhibitor and is noted for its sedative effect. Rarely it may cause priapism.
- *L-Tryptophan*: precursor of serotonin. Used in resistant depression as adjunct. Briefly withdrawn because of association with eosinophilia-myalgia syndrome. Available in UK on named patient basis.
- *Venlafaxine*: dual action antidepressant blocking re-uptake of both noradrenaline and serotonin. Less histaminergic, α adrenergic and cholinergic effects than TCAs. Like SSRIs, causes nausea upon commencing treatment. At high doses may cause marked hypertension in 10 per cent of subjects.
- *Viloxazine*: noradrenaline re-uptake inhibitor with few anticholinergic effects.
- *Zimeldine*: potent selective 5-HT uptake inhibitor. Withdrawn in 1983 after association with Guillain–Barré syndrome.
- *Mood stabilizers* such as lithium and *anticonvulsants* such as lamotrigine are used as antidepressants in particular in bipolar depression. Some *atypical antipsychotics* may also have antidepressant properties (olanzapine and quetiapine).
- *Antagonists at neurokinin* (NK_1) and *corticotropin-releasing factor* (CRF) *receptors* are currently in development and show promise.

SEROTONIN SYNDROME (SS)

Increasingly recognized since early 1990s, though reports exist from as early as 1955. Incidence unknown, probably due to wide spectrum in severity of presentation (severe reactions rare but potentially fatal). Most commonly seen with antidepressant polypharmacy (particularly irreversible MAOI + SSRI), or with insufficient washout between switching antidepressants (e.g. fluoxetine's metabolite norfluoxetine has a half-life ($t_{\frac{1}{2}}$) of 1 week; washouts of $5 \times t_{\frac{1}{2}}$ are recommended).

Can be caused by any drug(s) that $\uparrow$ net serotonin activity, particularly at $5\text{-}HT_{1A}$ and $5\text{-}HT_2$ receptors. Atypical antipsychotics may therefore be implicated, particularly if combined with serotonergic antidepressants. L-tryptophan augmentation significantly ↑ risk; lithium less so. Also associated with N-methyl-D-aspartate (NMDA) (ecstasy), tramadol, St John's Wort and sumatriptan. Risk factors: hypertension, atheroscleosis, hypercholesterolaemia.

Symptoms usually appear within a few hours of a medication change: mental state (confusion, agitation, hypomania, irritability), autonomic (sweating, pyrexia* >40°C, tachycardia), neurological (tremor, hyperreflexia, incoordination, myoclonus), GI (diarrhoea, nausea). Main differences from NMS are: hyperkinesia (as opposed to bradykinesia seen in NMS), presence of GI symptoms and relatively modest increases in serum CPK and possibly LFTs* compared with NMS.
(* tend to be associated with severe, potentially fatal cases).

[*SEROTOnIn*: **S**weating, **E**levated mood (mania) and mood change, **R**eflexes become brisk and can also get myoclonic jerks, **'O'**-tonomic instability – changes in heart rate, blood pressure etc., **T**emperature increases (pyrexia), c**ON**fusion, Gastro-**IN**testinal symptoms.]

MOOD STABILIZERS

LITHIUM

Lightest of alkali earth metals. Originally (1860s) used in treatment of gout, and not until almost a century later for the treatment of mania (Cade). Mechanism of action is incompletely understood; has little effect on EEG.

Rapidly absorbed following oral ingestion, reaching peak plasma levels within 2 hours. Complete absorption and distribution in total body water is achieved within 8 hours and subsequently it shifts slowly into cells. Lithium undergoes no protein binding or metabolism and is excreted unchanged in the urine. Available in liquid form (lithium citrate).

In acute mania, therapeutic plasma level is usually stated as 0.6–1.2 mmol/l. For prophylaxis, range is 0.4–0.8 mmol/l. Samples taken at 10 to 14 hours post-dose; ideal is 12 hours. Allow 5 to 7 days on same daily regime to establish level before taking a sample.

↑ monitoring required in pregnancy due to ante- and postnatal changes in plasma volume. ↑ fetal risk (up to 10 per cent teratogenicity), particularly cardiac problems in 1st trimester (such as Ebstein's anomaly). However, the absolute risk remains relatively low and must be weighed against the risk of relapse (which carries significant risk to the fetus) if medication is stopped.

Actions:

- ↓ neurotransmitter-mediated activation of second-messenger systems, probably via direct interaction with G-proteins, thus diminishing adenylate cyclase production of cAMP (NB: TSH (thyroid-stimulating hormone) stimulated release of T4 is cAMP-mediated, as is the effect of ADH on nephron permeability) and phosphoinositide metabolism
- neuronal membrane stabilization (slows repolarization by Na–K-ATPase).

Adverse effects of lithium:
- *Early*:
  - **T**iredness/fatigue: subjects often complain of feeling emotionally 'blunted'
  - **T**aste (metallic) → dysgeusia

- *T*hirst and dryness of mouth
- *T*remor (particularly noticeable in hands; propranolol may help)
- *Late*:
  - distal convoluted tubule resistance to ADH → nephrogenic diabetes insipidus
  - 2° hypothyroidism (see above) → goitre
  - weight gain
  - coarsening and loss of hair
  - oedema
  - hypokalaemia (may be associated with arrhythmias and T-wave flattening on ECG)
  - memory impairment
  - $10 \times \uparrow$ erythrocyte choline levels
  - leucocytosis
  - ↑ serotonergic transmission
  - ↓ central DA synthesis
  - exacerbates psoriasis
- *Toxic* (overdose plasma level >1.5 mmol/l):
  - diarrhoea
  - anorexia
  - dysarthria
  - ataxia
  - tinnitus
  - neurological damage (cerebellar syndrome)
  - vomiting
  - blurred vision
- *Severe toxicity* (level >2.5 mmol/l):
  - ↓ Coordination → Confusion → Convulsions → Circulatory failure → Collapse → Coma → Corpse
- *Factors that can lead to* *D*angerous toxicity:
  - *D*iuretics (thiazides; may ↑ Li^+ level by up to 25 per cent) and angiotensin-converting enzyme (ACE) inhibitors
  - *D*ietary *D*eficiency of Na^+: increases renal sodium, and hence lithium, retention
  - *D*ehydration: e.g. diarrhoea and vomiting, hot weather, exercise, polyuria etc.
  - *D*elivery: rapid postnatal ↓ plasma volume
  - NSAI*D*s
  - Acetazolamide (a carbonic anhydrase inhibitor used in epilepsy and to ↓ intra-ocular pressure) ↑ Li^+ excretion. Metronidazole ↑ risk of Li^+ toxicity during co-administration and for up to 3 weeks afterwards. Risk of neurotoxicity if Li^+ used with high doses of haloperidol (>20 mg/day).

CARBAMAZEPINE

An iminostilbene related to TCAs; acts by limiting the repetitive firing of sodium dependent action potentials. Used in the treatment of simple and complex partial seizures, and tonic–clonic seizures secondary to a focal discharge.

Additional indications: alternative or adjunctive mood stabilizer in lithium-resistant bipolar disorder, rapid cycling bipolar disorder, episodic dyscontrol syndrome/aggression, trigeminal neuralgia, panic attacks and atypical psychosis.

Induces CYP 3A liver enzymes, accelerating its own and many other drugs' metabolism, including the contraceptive pill (warn of need for extra contraception), anticoagulants and most antidepressants and antipsychotics. Also inhibits NA reuptake, and so is contraindicated for use with MAOIs. Relatively safe in pregnancy but remains potentially teratogenic.

Side-effects:

- dizziness ⎫ Carbamazepine has a linear dose–plasma concentration relationship.
- diplopia ⎬ These effects are dose related, and may be seen at therapeutic plasma
- ataxia ⎭ levels (4 to 12 μg/l).
- cognitive impairment
- headaches
- nausea, vomiting, constipation
- syndrome of inappropriate ADH secretion (SIADH)
- cholestatic jaundice (chemical rather than obstructive).

Effects from chronic use:

- hyponatraemia, eosinophilia
- liver failure.

Hypersensitivity:

- rashes (3 to 15 per cent, including lupus and Steven–Johnson syndrome)
- bone-marrow suppression ($\downarrow$ white cell count (WCC) predisposes to infection and $\downarrow$ platelets to bruising).

SODIUM VALPROATE

$\uparrow$ GABA neurotransmission and $\downarrow$ NA effect. Useful in the treatment of all forms of epilepsy. Increasingly used as first-line treatment for mania. Also used in treatment-resistant mania and rapid-cycling bipolar disorder. 'Depakote', or valproate semisodium, is a mixture of valproic acid and sodium valproate.

Potentially teratogenic (neural tube defect, heart anomalies and cleft lip); greatest risk in 1st trimester. $\uparrow$ Risk of neural tube defects partially compensated by supplementary folic acid (ideally started before pregnancy).

Dose-related adverse effects:

- irritability
- tremor
- weight gain
- intestinal irritation.

Effects from chronic use:

- alopecia
- amenorrhoea.

Hypersensitivity:

- hepatotoxicity
- pancreatic failure.

DRUGS USED IN THE TREATMENT OF ANXIETY

*AN*xiety is a central (brain) phenomenon involving the *A*mygdala (in the limbic system) and *N*A neurones in locus coeruleus (LC).

The major neurotransmitters (NT) involved in the mediation of anxiety are noradrenaline (NA), serotonin (5-HT) and gamma-aminobutyric acid (GABA) (the main inhibitory CNS neurotransmitter). Carbon dioxide and cholecystokinin (a neuropeptide in the amygdala) have also been implicated.

A somewhat over-simplified approach is that NA mediates the physical aspects of anxiety, and serotonin the mental aspects. However both these neurotransmitters, as well as both the physical and mental aspects of anxiety, are closely inter-related.

Noradrenergic neurons have α_1 (post-synaptic; widely implicated in side-effects of TCAs and neuroleptics) and α_2-receptors (pre- and post-synaptic). Pre-synaptic receptors are involved in the negative feedback of NA. Hence certain α-antagonists (e.g. yohimbine) can $\uparrow$ NA release = $\uparrow$ anxiety in susceptible individuals (e.g. those with panic disorder). Conversely, pre-synaptic α-agonists (e.g. clonidine) can/$\downarrow$ anxiety. β-receptor (post-synaptic) antagonists (e.g. propranolol) $\downarrow$ NA effect, and so $\downarrow$ anxiety symptoms (β-agonists such as salbutamol can have the opposite effect).

BENZODIAZEPINES (BZDs)

BZD-GABA receptor complexes comprise five subunits (which differ according to the particular receptor subtype) with a chloride channel in the middle. β-carbolines are endogenous ligands for these receptors, but their effect is complex.

BZDs potentiate the action of GABA by prolonging channel opening, causing $\uparrow$ hyperpolarization (influx of Cl^- ions) and so inhibiting depolarization (i.e. action potentials). They $\uparrow$ β and θ-wave activity on EEG, and have little effect in the absence of GABA (unlike barbiturates which can act independently of GABA), and so are relatively safe in overdose.

Type I BZD receptors are located in the cerebellum and are associated with sleep function. Type II and III receptors are located more in the spinal cord and limbic system, mediating the muscle relaxant and anxiolytic actions of BZDs.

Short half-life: hypnotic (i.e. sleep-inducing), e.g. temazepam (NB: a large amount may still act for a long time). Withdrawal problems more common. Initial $\downarrow$ REM sleep by 10–15 per cent, tolerance develops within 2 weeks.

Long half-life: anxiolytic, e.g. diazepam, chlordiazepoxide. Sometimes used as hypnotics (e.g. nitrazepam), which may lead to hangover and accumulation problems. Most commonly used in generalized and acute anxiety states. Treatment duration 2–4 weeks (as with hypnotics). Diazepam used in managing withdrawal from alcohol and short-acting BZDs; also absorbed rapidly and so used in suppressing seizures.

Flumazenil blocks the BZD–GABA receptor complex and can be given as an antidote in BZD overdose (NB: doses of >2 g have been survived). However, it has a short half-life and may need to be given several times as the subject repeatedly succumbs to the BZD in their system as each dose of flumazenil is metabolized.

Effects of benzodiazepines with increasing dose: ASHrAM (place of religious retreat). Anxiolytic → Sedative → Hypnotic → Anterograde Amnesia/Anticonvulsant/ Anaesthesia → Muscle-relaxant.

Adverse effects:

*D*ependence: recommended max. treatment duration 4 weeks

*D*rowsiness (daytime): esp. drugs with long half-lives

*D*ysarthria

*D*iplopia

*D*isorientation: 'paradoxical reaction' leading to hyperexcitability or delirium (especially in elderly).

Abrupt cessation after development of dependence (2–4 weeks of treatment) may lead to withdrawal symptoms:

'*S*tress' (anxiety, restlessness)

'*S*kinny' (nausea, ↓ appetite, weight loss)

'*S*trange' experiences (hypersensitivity, derealization/depersonalization, transient psychosis/perceptual distortions)

'*S*adness' (depressed mood)

*S*leep disturbance (rebound ↑ REM sleep with repeated waking)

*S*alivation

*S*weating

*S*exual disinterest

*S*haking (i.e. tremor)

*S*eizures.

No clear evidence that BZDs impair psychological adjustment, though some clinicians recommend avoiding them in bereavement. Relatively contraindicated in depression, chronic psychosis, phobic and obsessional states, breast-feeding and pregnancy (possible risk of congenital cleft palate and probable risk of respiratory depression in neonate). Absolutely contraindicated in respiratory depression and acute pulmonary insufficiency.

BZDs potentiate effects of:

- antidepressants
- analgesics (opioid)
- antihistamines
- alcohol
- antipsychotics (phenothiazines) and
- *d*isulfiram (by *d*ecreasing its *d*egradation).

Z-DRUGS

Zopiclone, zolpidem and zaleplon also act at the BZD–GABA receptor complex but at different sites to the BZDs. Originally marketed as being less addictive than BZDs, this has since been called into question. Indications/problems similar to that of BZDs.

Very short-half lives (minimal hangover, low accumulation), generally used for sleep induction (not sleep maintenance), acting mainly at the Type I BZD receptor.

BUSPIRONE

Partial 5-HT$_{1A}$ receptor agonist, weak D$_2$ receptor antagonist. Pre-synaptic action ↓ 5-HT release, post-synaptic activity ↑ 5-HT effect. Serotonergic activity returns to normal after 2 weeks of continuous use. Short half-life (3 hours; requires multiple doses daily) but available in slow-release form.

Improves symptoms of generalized anxiety disorder (GAD) over 1 to 2 months, particularly if there are associated depressive symptoms. 'Milder' anxiolytic than BZD and takes longer to act.

Main side-effects are nausea, headache, dizziness and sedation. No dependence syndrome/alcohol interaction.

PROPRANOLOL

A 'β-blocker': ↓ autonomic symptoms of anxiety (e.g. palpitations/tremor/tachycardia) by ↓ peripheral NA effect, interrupting the feedback mechanisms that can perpetuate and worsen anxiety. No proven direct psychological action, but fact that most other β-blockers appear to have little anxiolytic effect suggests an additional mechanism.

Relatively contraindicated in asthma, heart block/failure and poorly controlled diabetes. May be associated with bradycardia, hypotension, impotence, shortness of breath, depression, hallucinations, impaired short-term memory capacity, sleep disturbance and nightmares. Can cause rebound anxiety if stopped abruptly.

Also used to ameliorate tardive dyskinesia.

ANTIHISTAMINES

Hydroxyzine is a sedating antihistamine which can be used in the short-term management of anxiety. However, the evidence base for this indication is conflicting. Main side-effects are headache and sedation.

MEPROBAMATE

Introduced in 1955, meprobamate is a muscle relaxant that was used in the short-term management of anxiety. Due to problems with effectiveness, dependency and toxicity in OD, the *BNF* does not recommend its use.

ANTIDEPRESSANTS

All SSRIs (though only some are licensed and have trial evidence for this indication) and TCAs with serotonergic activity (e.g. clomipramine) can be of benefit in the treatment of the major anxiety disorders (generalized anxiety, agoraphobia, obsessive–compulsive disorder (OCD), panic disorder, post-traumatic stress disorder (PTSD) and social phobia) but not the specific phobias, with or without associated depressive symptoms. Additionally, MAOIs may be used in social phobia and venlafaxine in GAD.

In anxiety syndromes, SSRIs are generally titrated up from half their usual (i.e. anti-depressant) starting dose, and may take twice as long to have a clinical effect. Symptoms may worsen initially.

ANTIPSYCHOTICS

Most antipsychotics have an anxiolytic action. Chlorpromazine was widely prescribed in the management of anxiety, but this has now decreased. Trifluoperazine is sometimes used and is better than placebo at reducing anxiety after 4 weeks, but is associated with sedation and EPS.

ANTIEPILEPTICS

0.5 per cent of the general population has epilepsy, most commonly idiopathic. Treatment is mainly aimed at preventing further seizures (single seizures not treated). Incidence of epilepsy following a closed head injury 5 to 10 per cent (anterograde amnesia, loss of consciousness and the Glasgow Coma Scale (GCS) are valuable guides to functional prognosis); rises to 30 to 50 per cent in open injuries with brain laceration.

There is no specific 'epileptic personality', though epilepsy itself is positively associated with psychiatric disorders.

Many antiepileptics induce the metabolism of TCAs and the contraceptive pill. They also interact with each other (Table 14.1).

Table 14.1 Effect of antiepileptics used in combination

Effect of → on plasma levels of ↓	Carbamazepine enzyme inducer	Phenytoin enzyme inducer	Phenobarbitone enzyme inducer	Sodium valproate enzyme inhibitor
Carbamazepine		▼	▼	Δ
Phenytoin	▼Δ		▼Δ	▼Δ
Ethosuximide	↓	↓		↑
Sodium valproate	▲	▼	▼	
Phenobarbitone	▲	▲		▲
Primidone	▼	▼		▲
Clonazepam	▼	▼	▼	
Lamotrigine	▼	▼	▼	▲

↑ sometimes; ▲ significant effect; Δ smaller effect. Plasma monitoring is particularly important when these drugs are used in combination. NB primidone is largely converted to phenobarbitone.

CARBAMAZEPINE

See page 168

VALPROATE

See page 169

PHENYTOIN

A hydantoin; acts by limiting the repetitive firing of sodium-dependent APs. Useful in the treatment of all forms of epilepsy except absence seizures. It has a non-linear dose–plasma concentration curve and a narrow therapeutic index. Main teratogenic association is cleft palate; also implicated in neural tube defects. Cimetidine and fluoxetine may ↑ phenytoin level.

Dose-related adverse effects:

- dysarthria
- sedation
- ataxia.

Effects from chronic use:

- folate-deficient anaemia (megaloblastic)
- osteomalacia (pathological fractures)
- gingival hyperplasia
- facial features coarsen
- hypertrichosis
- cerebellar atrophy.

Hypersensitivity:

- rashes
- hepatitis.

Toxicity:

- ↑ seizure frequency
- tremor
- dizziness
- nystagmus.

ETHOSUXIMIDE

Possibly acts by hindering Ca^{2+} movement. Drug of choice in simple absence (petit mal) seizures. Excreted in breast-milk.

Dose-related adverse effects:

- anorexia
- sedation
- psychosis
- nausea and vomiting.

Hypersensitivity:

- bone marrow suppression (leucopenia)
- rashes.

PHENOBARBITONE

Barbiturate, acts by mimicking the effects of GABA. Indicated for use in all forms of epilepsy (except absence seizures). Secreted in breast-milk and may suppress sucking reflex in infant. Primidone is metabolized to phenobarbitone and is teratogenic.

Dose-related adverse effects:

- cognitive impairment
- ataxia (at therapeutic doses)
- sedation.

Effects from chronic use:

- megaloblastic anaemia (due to folate deficiency)
- osteoporosis because of inhibition of vitamin D absorption.

Hypersensitivity:

- rashes.

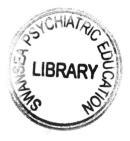

VIGABATRIN

γ-vinyl-substituted analogue of GABA; acts by inhibiting GABA aminotransferase. Indicated for use in chronic epilepsy not satisfactorily managed by other antiepileptics, and West's syndrome (infantile spasms).

Dose-related adverse effects:

- weight gain
- sedation
- depression.

Effects from chronic use:

- possible loss of peripheral vision.
- Has also been associated with psychosis.

LAMOTRIGINE

Inhibits the release of glutamate (the major excitatory amino acid in the CNS) through its action on sodium channels. Used as an adjunct in treatment-resistant partial and secondarily generalized tonic–clonic seizures, and those associated with Lennox–Gastaut syndrome. May be useful as an antidepressant in bipolar depression.

Dose-related adverse effects:

- ataxia
- diplopia

- vomiting
- headache.

Hypersensitivity:

- rashes
- hepatic dysfunction.

ANTIDEMENTIA DRUGS (FORMERLY NOOTROPICS*)

* Traditionally refers to oxiracetam, piracetam and pramiracetam: improved memory in animal models – possibly through metabolic enhancement. Limited efficacy in human dementia.

Acetylcholine (ACh) plays an important role in the neurobiology of memory. Drugs with anticholinergic action are associated with memory impairment (usually reversible) and confusion. Conversely, some drugs that enhance cholinergic action appear to boost cognitive function.

Cholinergic precursors: **lecithin or choline** Not effective.

Anticholinesterases (inhibit acetylcholinesterase breakdown of ACh) are used in treating the cognitive impairment of Alzheimer's disease (AD) and Lewy body dementia. They are indicated for mild to moderate dementia (the National Institute for Clinical Excellence (NICE) recommends a minimum starting Mini-Mental score of 13). Treatment for vascular dementia is aimed at the underlying cause (hypertension, diabetes etc.) and neuroprotection (e.g. calcium-channel blockers).

In AD, approximately 1/3 improve, 1/3 stabilize and 1/3 continue to deteriorate after 6 months on an anticholinesterase. Degree of benefit proportional to number of functioning cholinergic neurons; beneficial effect gradually tails off as disease progresses (most effective in early stages).

Donepezil (piperidine derivative, long $t_{1/2}$ [70 + hours] → once daily administration), **galantamine** (tertiary alkaloid, short $t_{1/2}$ [7 hours]) and **rivastigmine** (short $t_{1/2}$ [approx. 70 minutes]) are reversible anticholinesterases. The main side-effects of these drugs are dose-related to ↑ cholinergic activity and include GI problems (nausea, vomiting, diarrhoea), muscle cramps, urinary incontinence, dizziness and syncope. Other drugs such as NSAIDs, oestrogen and anti-oxidants may help delay the onset of AD.

Others not licensed in the UK. **Tacrine, velnacrine and metrifonate.** Tacrine is not licensed in the UK due to an association with hepatic toxicity.

GLUTAMATE ANTAGONIST

Memantine is an NMDA-receptor non-competitive antagonist used in the treatment of moderate to severe AD. NMDA receptors are acted upon by glutamate to mediate calcium entry into cells, which has been implicated in cell damage following neuronal injury. Side effects of confusion and hallucinations. Efficacy under evaluation.

MISCELLANEOUS TREATMENTS IN PSYCHIATRIC PRACTICE

PHYSICAL INTERVENTIONS

ELECTROCONVULSIVE THERAPY

The acute neurochemical effects of ECT are:

- ↑ activity of NA, DA and 5-HT
- ↓ activity of ACh.

There are corresponding changes of enzyme activity and metabolite concentrations. Chronic ECT application results in:

- ↑ 5-HT_2 (NB opposite to antidepressants), D_1 and adenosine A_1 purine receptor densities.
- ↓ β-adrenoceptor and muscarinic receptor densities.

There is also increased secretion of met-enkephalin, β-endorphin, vasopressin, ACTH and prolactin. Intriguingly, ECT may have neuroprotective effects via stimulation of neurogenesis (seen in animal studies).

Seizure threshold = the minimum charge required to induce a seizure. May vary considerably between individuals; most centres employ a system of stimulus dosing to determine the threshold.

ECT itself is a powerful anticonvulsant (hence successively need to ↑ dose to induce a seizure). Associated with memory impairment (usually temporary) but no clear evidence of brain damage. Occurrence of seizure is necessary for therapeutic effect, but length of seizure required is unclear.

Unilateral ECT (electrodes placed across one side of the head as opposed to bitemporal placement) is used to reduce possible cognitive impairment by inducing the seizure in the non-dominant hemisphere (though seizure will generalize), but requires a higher dose (i.e. charge, which is amps × seconds). Bifrontal electrode placement may also achieve the same.

Following ECT, patients experience an acute confusional state that lasts approximately 20 minutes. They can also experience difficulty in new learning (anterograde amnesia) that may last up to several months.

Contraindications to ECT treatment: recent stroke; raised ICP; recent MI with unstable rhythm.

PSYCHOSURGERY (associated with Moniz)

Only available in certain centres around the world. Used to treat intractable anxiety, depressive disorders and obsessive–compulsive disorder. Stereotactic procedures target the limbic system and its connections:

- stereotactic subcaudate tractotomy (SST)
- anterior capsulotomy
- cingulotomy
- limbic leucotomy.

All procedures associated with operative risks (haemorrhage, infection etc.) and cause an increase in the incidence of seizures (2 per cent).

VAGUS NERVE STIMULATION (VNS)

- Used in the treatment of more than 6000 people worldwide predominantly as a penultimate measure, prior to surgery, in the treatment of resistant partial-onset seizures in epilepsy.
- VNS exploits the fact that cranial nerves are direct extensions of the brain and as such have reciprocal influences on the limbic system and higher cortical activity.
- Vagus nerve is a mixed nerve and is largely afferent.
- Has been trialled in the treatment of depression with mixed results.
- Involves the placement of a subcutaneous bipolar pulse generator in the left chest wall that delivers electrical signals to an electrode wrapped around the vagus nerve in the neck.
- Common adverse effects include hoarseness, coughing and nausea.

DEEP BRAIN STIMULATION (DBS)

- Used in the treatment of Parkinson's disease (PD).
- Involves the delivery of a current using implanted electrodes.
- Mechanism of action is unknown.
- May have a role in the treatment of OCD.

TRANSCRANIAL MAGNETIC STIMULATION (TMS)

- Used widely for research and experimental focal stimulation of the brain. Can vary frequency, strength and site of stimulus.
- Current passed through coil induces current in cortex when TMS coil is placed adjacent to scalp.
- Can cause headaches, localized pain and auditory discomfort/damage. Risk of inducing a seizure (possible but rare).
- Trialled in the treatment of depression – with modest success.
- Being trialled in mania, schizophrenia and OCD.

ALCOHOL DEPENDENCE

Disulfiram is used to help prevent drinking alcohol by making the experience very unpleasant. It inhibits aldehyde dehydrogenase, leading to an accumulation of acetaldehyde (a metabolite of alcohol).

Disulfiram is metabolized to diethylthiocarbamate which inhibits DA-β-hydroxylase (catalyses DA $\rightarrow$ NA), leading to NA deficiency and an increase in DA. It also $\uparrow$ plasma levels of chlordiaxepoxide, flurazepam, diazepam and chlorazepate.

Disulfiram–ethanol reaction:

Vasodilatation (facial flush and drop in blood pressure)
Vomiting

Vertigo
Vision is blurred
Vicious headache
Visceral pains.

Avoid use in:

Asthma
Breathing difficulties
Cardiovascular disease
Diabetes
Elderly
Fitting (epilepsy, history of seizures)
Gravid (pregnant)
Hepatic disease.

Adverse effects of disulfiram:

*   gastrointestinal upset
*   halitosis
*   impotence
*   peripheral neuropathy
*   malaise
*   depression.

Acamprosate (taurine derivative) is used to help prevent craving in recovering alcoholics (doubles abstinence and increases 'time to first drink'). Believed to ↓ glutamate neurotransmission (action on NMDA receptor function possibly via effect on AMPA receptors). Contraindicated in severe liver damage.

Chlormethiazole/Clomethiazole (Heminevrin) is a sedative widely used in the elderly due to its short-half life (and therefore ↓ hangover). Also used in alcohol withdrawal, but is associated with dependency and can be mildly euphoric (and so abused).

Topiramate anticonvulsant drug acts via GABA – trialled unsuccessfully as a mood stabilizer. Used to improve drinking behaviour in alcohol dependence.

SMOKING

Bupropion (amfebutamone) is an antidepressant that has come to be used in helping alleviate nicotine addiction (Zyban). Thought to inhibit DA and NA re-uptake. ↑ Risk of seizures and contraindicated with history of eating disorders and bipolar disorder.

OPIOID DEPENDENCE

*   *Methadone*: an opioid agonist usually prescribed to substitute the use of heroin. Has a long half-life (can be given once daily) and does not give the 'rush' of acting drugs. Can be withdrawn gradually to prevent the onset of withdrawal symptoms.
*   *Naltrexone*: an opioid antagonist (non-selective action on δ, μ, κ receptors) that blocks the euphoric effects of opioids; used to prevent relapse. Also licensed as

maintenance treatment for recovered alcoholics, though effectiveness decreases with time. Contraindicated in liver failure/acute hepatitis.

- *Lofexidine*: reduces central sympathetic tone and offers symptomatic treatment of opioid withdrawal.
- *Buprenorphine*: an opioid partial agonist used in some centres as an alternative to methadone in those dependent on opioids.

ANTIMUSCARINIC DRUGS

Benzhexol, benztropine,* orphenadrine and **procyclidine*** are used in the treatment of parkinsonism. Not effective in the treatment of tardive dyskinesia (may actually exacerbate it). They should not be prescribed routinely. (* Can also be administered i.m. or i.v. and may be used in the emergency treatment of acute drug-induced dystonic reactions).

MISCELLANEOUS USES OF CERTAIN PSYCHOTROPICS

- *Tetrabenazine*: movement disorders (including tardive dyskinesia); Huntingdon's chorea. Depletes neuronal DA.
- *Imipramine*: childhood nocturesis.
- *Haloperidol*: motor tics; Gilles de la Tourette syndrome.
- *Haloperidol and chlorpromazine*: intractable hiccup.
- *Primidone*: essential tremor.
- *Pimozide, sulpiride and clonidine*: Gilles de la Tourette syndrome.
- *Desipramine*: craving in cocaine dependence.
- *Fluoxetine*: premature ejaculation.

PHARMACOKINETICS (what the body does to the drug)

ABSORPTION

The passage of a drug from its initial site of administration, through at least one membrane into the bloodstream. Determined by size, charge and lipid solubility of drug molecule as well as properties of absorption site (e.g. rate of blood flow; there is relatively poor muscle absorption in cardiac failure).

Administration may be enteral (oral, buccal, sublingual, rectal) or parenteral (intramuscular, subcutaneous, intravenous, intrathecal, topical, inhalational). Absorption may be avoided (e.g. intravenous route) or undesirable (e.g. certain topical applications).

Drugs administered enterally are subject to **first-pass metabolism** (except rectal), i.e. they are metabolized by the liver and gut mucosa prior to entering the systemic circulation (influenced by portal circulation, liver disease etc.). **Bioavailability** is the proportion of active drug that makes it into the systemic circulation.

The degree of ionization of a drug is determined by its dissociation constant and the pH of the ambient solution. Neutral molecules are much better absorbed than charged

Table 14.2

Route of administration and notes	Advantages	Disadvantages

Oral: absorption is mainly from small intestine by passive diffusion, pore filtration (most drugs too large) or active transport (specific)
Usually more appealing than injection
	Convenient
	Safe
	Allows more flexible
	  clinical management
	Gastric acidity
		Burden on patient to remember to
		  take medication
		Usually need food in stomach
		Less compliance and open to abuse/
		  misuse

Rectal: absorption from GI tract is influenced by gut motility, blood flow and area of absorption	Bypasses liver (1st-pass
	  metabolism)
	Bypasses stomach
	  (useful in nausea/
	  vomiting)
	Overcomes difficulty
	  of swallowing (e.g.
	  coma, seizure)
		Embarrassment
		
		Inflammation with frequent use

Intramuscular: better for lipid-soluble drugs	Depot treatment (slow
	  release), better compliance
	  and bioavailability
	Accurate knowledge of
	  drug use and less risk of
	  abuse
	Ensures regular clinical
	  contact
	Useful in emergencies
	No GI tract irritation
		Painful
		Risk of damage to nerves/vessels
		Risk of infection/abscess
		Delay in onset of side-effects and more
		  difficult to withdraw medication if
		  necessary

Intravenous	Rapid onset of action
	Can titrate dose and
	  response
	Avoids first-pass
	  metabolism
		Easy to overdose
		Infection, embolism, thrombosis
		Necrosis of tissues
		Injection into an artery

(i.e. ionized) ones, and so psychotropics are generally better absorbed from the intestine (which is relatively alkaline) than the stomach (where they are highly ionized).

DISTRIBUTION

The 'spreading out' of a drug between different body compartments (blood/intracellular/extracellular). Determined by:

- solubility of the drug and its extent of protein binding
- tissue permeability factors (pH partition, fat–water partition)
- haemodynamic factors
- partitioning membranes (blood–brain barrier, placenta).

Water forms 60–70 per cent of body weight: transcellular < plasma < interstitial < lipids < intracellular. Extracellular fluid (16 L) = blood plasma (5 L) + interstitial fluid (10 L) + lymph; intracellular fluid (30 L) total fluid in all cells of the body; transcellular fluid (1 L) peritoneal, synovial, pleural, intraocular, cerebrospinal fluids and digestive secretions.

The total amount of drug administered is usually greater than the amount that ends up in the plasma. The *volume of distribution* (V_d) is the volume of fluid necessary to dissolve the total amount of drug (D) in the body (i.e. the amount of drug administered) at a concentration equivalent to its concentration in the plasma (C_p). It is given by $V_d = D/C_p$.

The duration of action of a drug is inversely proportional to V_d. Body fat and high lipid solubility add to the V_d of a drug, which also increases with age because of a relative increase in body fat (although drug half-lives tend to ↑ with age due to changes in metabolism/excretion).

The brain contains neuronal and glial intracellular fluid; 200 mL of extracellular fluid and 110 mL of cerebrospinal fluid (approx. 20 mL is intraventricular and the remainder is in the subarachnoid space). In addition there is 80 mL of intracranial blood plasma (CSF pH is regulated independently from plasma pH).

Blood in brain capillaries is partitioned from the extracellular fluid compartment by the **blood–brain barrier** (BBB), which protects the brain by maintaining an exclusive environment. Certain substances readily cross the BBB – oxygen, carbon dioxide, glucose, some amino acids. It comprises (from brain → blood), important components *ABC*:

- glycoprotein and sialic acid neuronal surface covering
- perineuronal satellite cells (e.g. oligodendroglia)
- *A*strocyte end feet
- *B*asement membrane
- vessel wall
- *C*apillary endothelium (of brain and arachnoid + subarachnoid membranes).

Permeability is generally dependent upon lipid solubility. Most psychotropics are lipophilic and cross easily. Some substances require specific active transport mechanisms to cross (e.g. many amino acids). These transport systems are stereospecific for L-isomers.

The permeability of the BBB is increased by inflammation (e.g. mediated by histamine or some bacterial endotoxins) and anoxia-induced cerebral oedema.

The BBB is absent in some parts of the brain because of capillary vessel fenestration:

- hypothalamic regions, e.g. median eminence (allows releasing factors access to pituitary portal system)
- pineal body
- area postrema (vascularized strip of medullary tissue lying at caudal end of lateral border of 4th ventricle)
- choroid plexi
- hypophysis.

The placental barrier (between maternal and fetal vascular systems) also has a protective function. Substances cross by diffusion, active transport or pinocytosis. Lipid-soluble drugs cross more easily.

In the plasma, the competitive reversible binding of drugs to proteins (**protein binding**) is dependent upon:

- free drug concentration
- affinity of the drug for protein binding sites

- protein concentration (reduced in cardiac failure, renal/hepatic disease, carcinoma, malnutrition, burns).

Acidic drugs tend to bind to albumin; basic drugs (many psychotropics) bind to lipoprotein and α_1-acid-glycoprotein.

ELIMINATION

The processes by which drugs are broken down and removed from the body. The **clearance** is the rate at which a drug is eliminated and is given by $0.69 \times V_d/t_{1/2}$.

Biotransformation, the metabolism of drugs to produce more easily excreted products, is less necessary for small highly water-soluble molecules which may be excreted unaltered (e.g. lithium). It takes place principally in the liver, but also occurs in several other tissues: KILLS drug activity – Kidneys, Intestine, Lungs, Lymphocytes, Skin.

Hepatic biotransformation:

- *Phase I*: non-synthetic reactions such as oxidation, reduction and hydrolysis. The products may still be active. Oxidation is the commonest reaction and involves microsomal mixed-function oxidases (cytochrome p450 isoenzymes), located on smooth endoplasmic reticulum.
- *Phase II*: generally drugs that undergo non-synthetic reactions require further processing prior to elimination. This involves conjugation (synthetic reactions), whereby the drug is chemically coupled (conjugated) to a water-soluble molecule (such as glucuronate; glutathione; glycine; glutamine; acetate; sulphate). The resulting conjugate is water soluble and so can be excreted in urine or bile.

Most drugs undergo first-order kinetics, i.e. the rate of metabolism is proportional to the amount of drug. Alcohol (metabolized by isoenzyme CYP 2E1) and phenytoin (CYP 2C9, which also metabolizes warfarin) have a zero-order kinetic profile; they are metabolized at a constant rate irrespective of the amount of drug.

The enzymes involved in biotransformation can be **induced** by the action of certain drugs, increasing their activity. This can affect the plasma concentration of the drug itself (auto-induction, e.g. carbamazepine) and/or that of other drugs. Conversely, enzyme inhibition slows enzymatic activity, and may or may not be of benefit (e.g. MAOIs, phenothiazines and butyrophenones ↑ levels of TCAs).

Most drugs and their metabolites undergo renal excretion. This is affected by nephron function (as measured by the glomerular filtration rate, GFR) and the drug's plasma concentration, solubility, protein binding and molecular weight (MW < 300 → kidney, >300 → bile).

Excretion also occurs in: bile, faeces, saliva, sweat and milk. Biliary excretion of some substances is active and even when a substance has been excreted into the intestine it may be reabsorbed (entero-hepatic cycle). Elimination of drugs via breast-milk is not significant quantitatively but is important with respect to potential toxic effects on a breast-feeding infant. Milk is of lower pH than plasma and can concentrate certain substances.

Genetics

15

DNA AND RNA

nucleo*S*ide = nitrogenous base (e.g. adenine) + *S*ugar (ribose or deoxyribose)
nucleo*T*ide = nucleoside + phospha*T*e.

DNA (DEOXYRIBONUCLEIC ACID)

Large polymer found in chromosomes of cell nucleus and mitochondria. Linear backbone consists of successive 5-carbon sugar residues (deoxyribose) linked by covalent 3′,5′ **phosphodiester bonds**. Four nucleotides (purines; **adenine** [A] and **guanine** [G] and pyrimidines; **cytosine** [C] and **thymine** [T]) form two strands that are arranged in a **double helix (DNA duplex)**. The hydrogen bond **complementary** base-pairing between the two **anti-parallel** strands is always A–T and G–C (2 and 3 hydrogen-bonds respectively in each **base pair**) in accordance with **Chagraff's rule**. Hydrogen bonds can be disrupted by changes of pH or heat.

RNA (RIBONUCLEIC ACID)

Same structure as DNA but contains ribose instead of deoxyribose and uracil [U] instead of thymine.

There are several kinds of RNA: messenger RNA (**mRNA**), ribosomal RNA (**rRNA**), transfer RNA (**tRNA**) and heterogenous nuclear RNA (**hnRNA**).

DNA REPLICATION

The process of DNA synthesis commences with **helicase** unwinding the DNA duplex, giving rise to a **replication fork**. Synthesis can only occur in the direction 5′ → 3′. Along one strand, designated the **leading strand**, replication occurs in the direction of movement of the replication fork, and so can be carried out continuously as the DNA unwinds (using **DNA polymerase δ**). Along the other strand, called the **lagging strand**, 5′ → 3′ synthesis (using **DNA polymerase α**) creates pieces of DNA called **Okazaki fragments**, which are then joined together by **DNA ligase** (semi-continuous synthesis).

DNA replication is described as **semi-conservative** because each strand directs the synthesis of a complementary one, leading to two identical daughter duplexes. Each new duplex contains a new strand and one original (i.e. conserved) strand. Complete DNA replication takes approximately 8 hours.

GENES

The human genome contains about 100 000 human genes.

Gene: DNA segment that encodes for a function-specific protein/set of proteins.

Chromosomal pairs contain two copies of any particular gene (maternal and paternal), known as **alleles**. If the two alleles are the same the individual is described as being **homozygous** for that gene; if they are different the individual is **heterozygous**.

Genotype: the coded genetic make-up of an individual.

Phenotype: the expressed genetic make-up of an individual.

A *dominant* gene is expressed in the phenotype even if only present on one chromosome.

A *recessive* gene is only expressed in those that are homozygous for that gene.

Genes make up 1 per cent of human DNA. The remainder is thought to be involved in regulatory and supportive processes. Within genes there is DNA that does not code for amino acids. These segments are called *introns* (they remain *in*side the nucleus). *Exons* are transported into the cytoplasm and code for amino acids, i.e. they are *ex*pressed (**coding DNA**). Three nucleotide bases form a **codon** and denote a specific amino acid. Spliceosomes (nuclear organelles) splice exons into mRNA and remove introns from heterogenous RNA.

GENE EXPRESSION

The flow of genetic information is largely unidirectional from DNA to RNA to polypeptides. This is known as the **central dogma of molecular biology**. Gene expression follows the **colinearity principle** and involves **transcription** and **translation**. Only some of the RNA created by transcription is then translated into polypeptide/protein.

TRANSCRIPTION

Transcription proceeds $5' \rightarrow 3'$ and the initial step involves production of a complementary RNA transcript. Only one of the DNA strands acts as a template (**template strand/antisense strand**). The RNA transcript has the same orientation ($5' \rightarrow 3'$) and base sequence (but with U replacing T) as the non-template strand, and so is called the **sense strand**. In addition to its structural and coding components (introns/exons), a typical gene consists of a transcription regulatory site, a promotor region that 'prepares' for transcription (e.g. TATA, GC and CAAT 'boxes'), and a transcription initiation site. Transcription involves **RNA polymerases** (types I, II and III; most genes encode peptides and are transcribed by RNA polymerase II) and a variety of transcription factors.

Post-transcriptional processing involves RNA splicing, capping and polyadenylation.

- *RNA splicing*: introns are removed by endonucleolytic cleavage at specific **splice junctions** from the **primary transcript** (transcription of complete gene) by **spliceosomes**.
- *Capping*: RNA polymerase II transcripts undergo the addition of a specialized nucleotide to the 5′ end of mRNA. This is thought to help RNA splicing, aid mRNA transport into the cytoplasm, protect the mRNA transcript from enzymatic degradation and facilitate ribosomal attachment.
- *Polyadenylation*: following transcript cleavage the mRNA 3′ end is polyadenylated (approx. 200 adenylate residues are added) 15–30 nucleotides downstream of the AAUAAA element. This is thought to add stability, aid mRNA transport into the cytoplasm and facilitate translation.

TRANSLATION

Once transported out of the nucleus into the cytoplasm, mRNA undergoes translation by ribosomes that then organize, with the use of tRNA, the appropriate amino acids to form the designated peptide. Mitochondria also contain ribosomes and are capable of protein synthesis.

In most cases the **initiation codon** AUG (which specifies methionine) initiates translation. Each tRNA, carrying a specific amino acid, has a trinucleotide sequence (the **anticodon**) that matches the relevant codon on the mRNA. Hence, complementary base pairing takes place between the RNAs, and the correct amino acid is inserted into the growing peptide chain.

Peptidyl transferase catalyses a condensation reaction between the *a*mino group of amino acid being *a*dded and the *c*arboxyl group of the amino acid in the *c*hain, resulting in successive peptide bonds. Linear translation of mRNA continues until a **termination codon** is encountered.

The initial polypeptide often undergoes **post-translational modification**. This includes the addition of certain groups [methylation (CH_3), phosphorylation (PO_4^-), hydroxylation (OH), carboxylation (COOH), acetylation (CH_3CO) and glycosylation)] and internal cleavage. Many polypeptides are synthesized as precursors containing an N-terminal **signal/leader sequence**. This is usually necessary for transmembrane transport of the polypeptide.

The genetic code is described as being **degenerate** as there are many more codons ($4^3 = 64$) than amino acids (20). Many amino acids are therefore specified by several codons. However, some are only specified by a single codon, e.g. tryptophan and methionine.

CHROMOSOMES

Human somatic cell nuclei contain **46** chromosomes; 22 pairs of **autosomal chromosomes** (44 autosomes) and one pair of **sex chromosomes**. Similar autosomes are paired and termed **homologous**; however, they are not identical.

Specialized sex cells (**gametes**) have half the number of chromosomes (23) and are termed **haploid**, as opposed to somatic cells which are described as **diploid**. A normal male is therefore 44XY and a normal female 44XX.

Gametes arise from specific gonadal somatic cells which undergo reductive cell division termed **meiosis**. The fusion of two haploid cells produces diploid somatic cells, as does binary cell division, which includes **mitosis** (nuclear division) and **cytokinesis** (cytoplasmic division).

Differentiation of somatic cells can alter their DNA, and some have no chromosomes at all (platelets, red blood cells) whereas others are multinucleated (muscle cells). Additional DNA duplication prior to cell division (**endomitosis**) results in **polyploid** cells which have additional sets of chromosomes (hepatocytes, megakaryocytes).

Chromatin: the basic material of chromosomes (CR), consisting of DNA complexed with proteins. DNA is tightly packaged to form **nucleosomes** which consist of a central core of **histone proteins** around which 146 base pairs of double-stranded DNA are coiled. Successive nucleosomes are linked by spacer DNA and the nucleosomes themselves are further coiled to form a **chromatin fibre**. Chromatids consist of coiled loop-scaffold complexes, in which chromatin fibre loops are attached to a central scaffold protein such as topoisomerase II.

CRs are normally very thin and drawn out. Therefore they are usually examined during mitosis or meiosis when they are condensed.

Karyotype: an individual's set of CRs. Preparation involves:

- cell division arrest, dispersion, fixing and staining of CRs
- CRs are then photographed and arranged according to their identity.

The number of X CRs in a somatic cell nucleus can be determined without karyotyping. The number of **chromatin bodies** (**Barr bodies**, BB) equals the number of X CRs minus one. (Chromatin body number = No. of X CRs − 1; e.g. XX female = 1 BB.)

Each CR has a constricted region that is prominent during mitosis and meiosis. This is called the **centromere** and it divides CRs into two arms of differing lengths.

The long arm is designated **q**, the short arm is designated **p**.

The positioning of the centromere gives rise to **metacentric** CRs (centromere central) and **acrocentric** CRs (centromere nearer one end).

The staining of CRs produces bands that are then ascribed names and numbers. This produces a **chromosomal map**.

Standardized designation: e.g. **Xq28**

> First character (**X**) can be letter (X or Y) or number (1–22) specifying the CR
> Second character (**q**) specifies short or long CR arm (p or q)
> Third character (**2**) designates particular CR region
> Fourth character (**8**) identifies band

CELL DIVISION

*M*itosis (*M* phase) is a relatively short stage which alternates with the **interphase**. Interphase is a much longer period and consists of three phases: a gap between the M and S phases (**G1** phase), the *s* phase itself, during which DNA is Synthesized, and another subsequent gap (**G2** phase) between the S and M phase to complete the cycle. Cells that are non-dividing remain in stage G0 (a modification of G1), and only those cells that are committed to cell division enter the S phase.

MITOSIS

Somatic cell nuclear division: five phases: *DIP*lo*MAT*

*D*ivision =
*I*nterphase
*P*rophase
*M*etaphase
*A*naphase
*T*elophase.

MEIOSIS

Reproductive cells undergo two stages of cell division resulting in haploid gametes. The stages of mitosis are then repeated with the exception of the interphase.

INHERITANCE

Gregor Mendel, Austrian monk and botanist: Mendelian inheritance applies to single gene defects (deletions, inversions, insertions). Capital letter denotes dominant allele, lower case denotes recessive allele (see Table 15.1).

Table 15.1 Mendelian inheritance

Parents	DDDD × dddd	DDdd × DDdd	DDMM × ddmm
Offspring (F₁)	Dd	DD:Dd:Dd:dd	DdMm
Offspring (F₂)			DDMM, DDMm, ddmm etc.
Law of …	Uniformity	Segregation	Independent Assortment
Mendel's		First Law	Second Law

INHERITANCE OF DISEASE

Autosomal dominant: dominant allele leads to manifestation of disease in all individuals that possess it. Hence shows 'vertical' transmission as phenotypic trait is evident in every generation. Affects both sexes equally. Degree of penetrance and expressivity cause variance of clinical features. Spontaneous occurrence of autosomal dominant disorder may be due to a new mutation.

Autosomal recessive: expression of disease requires that individual carries two alleles (i.e. is homozygous). Heterozygous individuals carry but do not phenotypically manifest the disease, and hence the disease seems to miss generations and give the appearance of horizontal transmission. Rare disorders raise the likelihood of consanguineous parents.

X-linked disorders: affected allele on X chromosome. Transmission between males is not possible (only mother → son). Can be **dominant** (affected allele is dominant) or **recessive** (affected allele is recessive and all males with affected allele manifest the disorder. Females if heterozygous are carriers).

GENETIC STUDIES

CONVENTIONAL METHODS

Family studies: these compare rates of a disorder in proband's (i.e. affected individual's) relatives (first and second degree) and general population. First degree relatives (biological parents, siblings and offspring) share 50 per cent of genome. Second degree relatives (grandparents, uncles, aunts, nieces, nephews and grandchildren) share 25 per cent of genome.

Disadvantages:

- common environment (hence need for twin/adoption studies)
- varying ages of relatives. Disease may not have yet presented.

(Clinically, increased incidence/prevalence is seen in relatives of those with *a*nxiety neurosis, *a*norexia nervosa, *a*lcoholism, Alzheimer's disease, and *a*utistic disorder.)

Twin studies: comparison of rates of disorder in co-twins of probands. Monozygotic (identical) twins have same genome. Dizygotic (fraternal) twins share 50 per cent of genome. Monozygotic twins at greater genetic risk.

Concordance rate: rate of disorder in proband co-twin. Can be derived according to pairs (concordant sets of twins/total no. of twin sets) or probands (proband co-twins with concurrent disorder/total no. of co-twins).

Concordance rate is generally more suitable when examining discrete traits; correlation coefficient is better for continuous traits.

Disadvantages:

- assortative mating (↑ rate of illness in dizygotic twins relative to monozygotic twins)
- age correction measures and sampling may introduce bias
- twins more susceptible to injury at birth and more likely to have congenital abnormalities.

Adoption studies: individual is adopted away from biological parents and reared by unrelated adoptive parents. Studies can centre on the adoptee or the whole adoptee family and can also use monozygotic twin adoptees to enhance their power.

Cross-fostering is a complicated method that is occasionally used: adopted children of affected biological parents are compared with the children of biologically unaffected parents adopted by affected parents. If the rate of disorder in parents is studied, this is known as an adoptee family study.

Disadvantages:

- time consuming
- difficult to find appropriate cases (criteria difficult to fulfil)
- adoption process is not necessarily random
- data concerning biological parents may not be available
- confounding psychological influence of being adopted.

EXPERIMENTAL METHODS

The main ways to locate particular genes possibly implicated in the aetiology of a disorder are **linkage** and **association** studies.

Recombination occurs through the 'crossover' of genetic material between homologous pairs of chromosomes. It is the creation of new chromosomes by swapping maternal and paternal versions of the same genes (i.e. alleles). The closer the alleles are on an individual chromosome the less likely they are to be separated during meiosis, thus maintaining their relative position on the new (mixed) chromosome.

Note that in such instances recombination is said not to have occurred (for these particular alleles). Instead, the genes are usually inherited together and so described as being genetically linked. The distance between two alleles can be approximated from the number of siblings (i.e. individuals with the same parents) in whom recombination of the two alleles has occurred.

The **recombinant fraction** (θ) is a measure of the frequency with which this recombination occurs. It is expressed as a fraction, ranging from 0 (i.e. no recombination, and the genes are not separated) to 0.5 (the genes are sufficiently distant for independent assortment to occur, i.e. the genes are separated and inherited independently).

The odds of there being linkage for a particular recombinant fraction versus there being no linkage can be expressed as an odds ratio. The logarithm of this ratio is defined as the **LOD score** (log of odds). A LOD score of -2 or less excludes linkage, and a score of 3 or more is taken as evidence of linkage (with single-gene Mendelian inheritance).

Restriction endonucleases are enzymes that cleave DNA. Acting at specific nucleotide sequences, they produce many small DNA fragments of varying length called **restriction fragment length polymorphisms** (RFLPs). These form a unique pattern that differs between people and undergoes Mendelian inheritance. **Gene probes** are DNA pieces produced with complementary nucleotide sequences, enabling them to hybridize with specific portions of the genome.

Polymorphisms at cleavage sites result in fragments. These can be identified using **Southern blotting** and certain DNA probes.

Linkage analysis uses DNA markers such as RFLPs to find an association between them and a particular disease or illness locus. If there is a departure from independent assortment ($\theta < 0.5$) then linkage is inferred.

PHARMACOGENETICS/PHARMACOGENOMICS/PSYCHOPHARMACOGENOMICS

Broadly encompasses: molecular approaches applied to individual variation in response to drug treatments.

Everyone responds differently to the same dose of the same medication depending upon age, psychological factors (hence placebo effect), renal and hepatic function, drug interactions and genetic factors. Pharmacogenetics is concerned with the role of genetic factors in predicting both drug response and potential adverse effects.

Pharmacogenomics is a non-hypothesis-based approach that examines the relationship between whole genome factors and drug response at various levels (cellular, tissue, and individual or treatment group). It will have a significant impact on drug discovery, design, and clinical application.

MULTIFACTORIAL BEHAVIOURAL DISORDERS

Approximately 50 per cent of the variation seen in major behavioural disorders in the population results from differences in shared genes. Complex behaviour appears to be determined by a wide range of factors, some of them genetic and some environmental. Genetic factors individually contribute only a small amount, however; by acting in conjunction with environmental triggers they potentially have an enormous impact on the final phenotype. Consequently these are referred to as quantitative trait loci (QTLs).

METHODS OF BEHAVIOURAL GENE HUNTING

- *Coordinated pathway genotype analysis*: enables simultaneous survey of several genes and has successfully detected potential gene variants associated with anxiety and depression. When coupled with life event data has identified the need to include environmental measures in association studies. Depression (in males and females) and antisocial behaviour (in males) have been linked to low-transcription variants of neurotransmitter genes (serotonin transporter and monoamine oxidase, respectively) – in individuals subjected to stressful early life environments.
- *Genome-wide linkage scans*: extend search beyond candidate genes and employ linkage or association strategies. Linkage is systematic but not powerful. Using approximately 400 markers it is possible to search the genome for genes influencing a behavioural disorder, with each marker scanning up to ten million base pairs for a gene of large effect. Linkage can identify chromosomal regions harbouring potential candidate genes; however, it is inefficient at detecting genes of small effect.
- *Genome-wide association studies*: seek allelic association between marker alleles and population traits as opposed to within families. More powerful for detecting QTLs of small effect. New microarray technology may allow the detection of QTLs of small effect size that contribute to major behavioural disorders.

PSYCHIATRIC DISORDERS

SCHIZOPHRENIA

Familial aggregation of schizophrenia has been shown in family, twin and adoption studies.

Lifetime risk of schizophrenia in relatives of schizophrenic proband is shown in Table 15.2.

Modes of inheritance

Single major locus (no such locus has been found), **polygenic** and **multifactorial**.

Mixed model is also proposed, with major gene operating against multifactorial background.

Linkage studies: implicate several genes. None replicated or sufficiently supported. (5q; 11q; 6p-HLA9).

Association with velocardiofacial syndrome involving chromosome C22q.

Table 15.2 Lifetime risk of schizophrenia in relatives (general population 1%)

Relation to proband	Lifetime risk (%)
Parent	6
Sibling (including dizygotic (DZ) twin)	10
Sibling (with a parent also affected)	17
Children	13
Children (both parents affected)	46
Grandchildren, half siblings	4
Uncles, aunts, nephews, nieces	3
Monozygotic (MZ) twin	46

Candidate genes that are postulated to be associated with schizophrenia include:

* dysbindin,
* neuregulin,
* G72/D-amino acid oxidase,
* proline dehydrogenase (PRODH),
* regulator of G protein signalling (RGS-4),
* catechol-O-methyltransferase (COMT),
* 5-HT$_{2A}$ receptor,
* dopamine D$_3$ receptor,
* PPP3CC.

These need to be studied a great deal more; however, 'schizophrenia genes' are emerging as likely.

AFFECTIVE DISORDERS

Family studies: first degree relatives of unipolar depressives have an increased risk of unipolar depression. First degree relatives of bipolar patients have an increased risk of both unipolar and bipolar illness.

Twin studies: monozygotic:dizygotic concordance ratio is approximately 2:1 for unipolar disorder and 4:1 for bipolar disorder.

Adoption studies:

* 26 per cent of biological parents of bipolar patients have mood disorder
* 28 per cent of biological parents of bipolar adoptees have mood disorder
* 12 per cent of adoptive parents of bipolar adoptees have mood disorder.

Linkage studies: some familial links of bipolar illness to glucose-6-phosphate deficiency and colour blindness (Xp).

Also in some pedigrees linkage to chromosome 11. However, results lack replication. Gene complex **G72/G30** strongly implicated in bipolar disorder.

Evidence is also emerging that points to 12p, 14p, and 15p as chromosomal regions potentially containing genes related to bipolar disorder.

ALCOHOLISM

Family studies: runs in families. Relatives of alcoholics more likely to be alcoholics.

Twin studies: concordance in monozygotic twins higher than that for dizygotic twins.

Adoption studies: parental alcoholism increases risk of alcoholism in males ($\times$4).

NARCOLEPSY

Monozygotic concordance of 17–36 per cent, with 1–2 per cent first degree proband relatives affected (representing a 20–40× increase over general population). Thought to be caused through deficient hypocretin (also called orexin) effect, either due to a loss of hypocretin cells or of hypocretin receptors.

Hypocretin is an excitatory neuropeptide found in the lateral, posterior and peri-fornical hypothalamus. Extensive cortical and sub-cortical projections, impinging on the noradrenergic, histaminergic, serotonergic and dopaminergic systems. Stimulates appetite and wakefulness, and has a regulatory role in neuroendocrine functioning.

Strong association between narcolepsy and the human leukocyte antigen DR2 (specifically HLA allele DQB1*0602), implicating an autoimmune process. However, clear polymorphism of the relevant genes is very rare, despite 85 per cent of narcoleptics manifesting ↓ CSF hypocretin levels.

OTHERS

There is a significant genetic contribution to the familial aggregation of:

- phobia
- social phobia (risk to relatives ×3)
- panic disorder (risk to relatives ×10)
- obsessive–compulsive disorder
- eating disorders.

GENETIC ABNORMALITIES AND BIRTH DEFECTS

One in forty pregnancies result in the birth of a child with a congenital abnormality. The cause of most is unknown. The aetiology can be genetic, environmental or multi-factorial.

- *Environmental factors*:
  - maternal factors (prior to and during pregnancy and at the time of birth)
  - maternal illness (e.g. diabetes)
  - infections (toxoplasmosis, rubella, cytomegalovirus, herpes)
  - medications, drugs and toxins (e.g. ethanol, heavy metals, phenytoin)
  - mechanical factors (e.g. forceps delivery)
  - radiation (X-rays)
  - pollution.
- *Genetic disorders*:
  - chromosomal abnormalities
  - numerical changes (increase or absence)
  - structural changes (deletions and translocations)
  - single gene abnormalities
  - autosomal (dominant and recessive)
  - sex chromosome linked (dominant and recessive).
- *Multifactorial.*

CHROMOSOMAL ABNORMALITIES

Disorders result from:

- a change in the number of chromosomes
- change in chromosomal structure; deletion/loss, addition
- **translocation** of chromosomal material between chromosomes.

5 per cent of fetuses have chromosomal abnormalities and of these 90 per cent abort. 0.5 per cent of live newborn infants have chromosomal abnormalities (autosomal:sex CRs; 2:1).

AUTOSOMAL ABNORMALITIES

Down's syndrome

Described by Langdon Down in 1866. It is a common cause of mental retardation.

Few with Down's syndrome have an IQ >50, and of all those with IQ <50 one-third have Down's syndrome.

Maternal age is an important risk factor:

risk at age   *20* years   1:*20*00

                     45 years   1:*45*

Overall incidence 1:*66*0 live births.

95 per cent of cases due to meiotic non-disjunction (trisomy 21), i.e. failure of chromosomal separation, producing a gamete with an extra chromosome. 4 per cent due to translocation of genetic material between chromosome 21 and another. In 1 per cent of cases only a proportion of the cells have trisomy and the remainder are normal (mosaic).

The risk of recurrence with non-disjunction is about 1 per cent, in cases of translocation the risk is much higher.

Stigmata:

- *Eyes*: **BCDEF**
  - **B**rushfield's spots
  - **C**ataracts and conjunctivitis
  - **D**eviation (squint)
  - **E**picanthic folds and ectropion
  - **F**issure (palpebral) upwardly slanting.
- *Head*:
  - small, brachycephalic skull with flat occiput
  - small rounded ears
  - high cheekbones
  - large fissured tongue.
- *Body*: **BCDEFGH**
  - **B**owel disorder (Hirschsprung's disease)
  - **C**ryptorchidism
  - **D**uodenal atresia
  - **E**ndocardial cushion defects (40–50 per cent)
  - straight **F**ollicles (pubic hair)
  - poor development of external **G**enitalia
  - umbilical **H**ernia.

- *Hands and feet*:
  - single palmar crease (simian) (50 per cent)
  - clinodactyly (50 per cent)
  - abnormal dermatoglyphics
  - broad hands and short stubby fingers
  - short, broad feet
  - large cleft between 1st and 2nd toes.
- *Brain*:
  - epilepsy [10 per cent]
  - mental retardation
  - earlier development of senile plaques (early onset Alzheimer's disease)
  - marked $\uparrow$ P300 latency.
- *General*:
  - hypotonia
  - leukaemia (1 per cent)
  - hypothyroidism (3 per cent)
  - short stature.

Edward's syndrome (trisomy 18)
95 per cent of fetuses abort. Main cause non-disjunction.
 Overall incidence 1:3000 live births. 30 per cent die within one month. Maternal age effect.
 Stigmata:

- mental retardation
- craniofacial abnormalities: micrognathia, prominent occiput, low-set fawn-like ears
- palmar crease, abnormal dermatoglyphics and when hand is clenched overlapping fifth and index fingers
- rocker-bottom feet
- short sternum
- cardiac and renal malformations
- cryptorchidism (males).

Patau's syndrome (trisomy 13)
Overall incidence 1:7600 live births. Virtually all die by age 3 years (50 per cent within one month). Maternal age effect.
 Stigmata:

- cleft lip/palate
- polydactyly
- ophthalmic defects
- low-set ears.

Cri-du-chat syndrome
Deletion on short arm of chromosome 5.
 Overall incidence 1:50 000 live births. More common in females than males.
 Stigmata:

- mental retardation
- abnormal cry

- spasticity
- craniofacial abnormalities: microcephaly, 'moon-faced', epicanthic folds, hypertelorism and alert expression.

Prader–Willi syndrome

Overall incidence 1:15 000 live births. Partial deletion of long arm of chromosome 15 (chromosomal derivation usually paternal).

Stigmata: *PRADER*

- *P*alpebral fissures – almond shaped
- *R*ound face
- *A*ngry outbursts
- *D*own-turned mouth
- *E*at excessively (hyperphagia)
- *R*educed tone (infantile hypotonia)
- Small: in height; hands and feet; testicles.

Retinoblastoma

Deletion on CR 13.

Overall incidence 1:20 000 live births.

Stigmata:

- bilateral retinoblastoma
- reduced IQ.

Wilms' tumour (renal)

Deletion on CR 11.

Overall incidence 8 cases per million children.

Stigmata:

- *I*Q reduced
- *I*rises are absent (aniridia)
- *I*ndeterminate (ambiguous) genitalia.

SEX CHROMOSOME ABNORMALITIES

Kleinfelter's syndrome

Overall incidence 1:500. Phenotypic male has extra X chromosome(s) (maternal in 60 per cent cases). Usually 47XXY. 15 per cent are mosaics. Maternal age effect.

Stigmata:

- infertility (usual mode of presentation)
  - small testis (<2 cm length)
  - low testosterone levels
  - poorly developed secondary sexual characteristics
- gynaecomastia
- variable degree of mild mental retardation (often normal)
- elongated limbs (disproportionate body).

Associations: diabetes, osteoporosis, emphysema, scoliosis, breast cancer, schizophrenia.

47XYY

Overall incidence 1:700. Phenotypic males have extra Y chromosome because of paternal YY sperm.
   Stigmata:

- very tall (body proportions normal)
- IQ slightly lower than normal.

   Doubtful associations with aggression and criminality.

Extra X chromosomes

XXX, XXXX etc. very mild abnormalities with a single additional X chromosome; however, with each additional X chromosome degree of mental retardation becomes more evident.

Turner's syndrome

Overall incidence 1:2500 (female births). Diagnosed by buccal mucosal cell chromosomal analysis. XO. Barr body.
   60 per cent are 45X.
   Remainder are deletions of X chromosome long/short arm or mosaics.
   Life-span and intelligence are normal.
   Stigmata:

- short stature
- craniofacial abnormalities:
  - webbed neck
  - micrognathia
  - low hair-line (back of head)
  - downward slanting palpebral fissures
  - down-turned mouth
  - low-set ears
- limb and truncal abnormalities:
  - lymphoedema
  - cubitus valgus (wide carrying angle)
  - wide separation of nipples (broad, shield-like chest)
- ovarian dysgenesis (streak ovaries): infertility
- cardiovascular defects:
  - atrial septal defects
  - coarctation of the aorta
  - hypertension
- Hashimoto's thyroiditis.

SINGLE GENE ABNORMALITIES

AUTOSOMAL DOMINANT DISORDERS

- Huntingdon's disease
- Phacomatoses (tuberose sclerosis, neurofibromatosis, Sturge–Weber syndrome, von Hippel–Lindau syndrome)

- Acrocephalosyndactyly (Apert's syndrome)
- Craniofacial dysostosis (Crouzon's syndrome)
- Mandibulofacial dysostosis (Treacher Collins' syndrome)
- Wardenburg syndrome
- Myotonic distrophy.

AUTOSOMAL RECESSIVE DISORDERS

Metabolic disorders
- Fat metabolism:
  - Niemann-Pick disease
  - Tay–Sachs disease
  - Gaucher's disease
- Protein metabolism:
  - phenylketonuria
  - Hartnup disease
- Mucopolysaccharidoses:
  - Hurler's syndrome
  - Hunter's syndrome
- Carbohydrate metabolism:
  - galactosaemia.

OTHERS

- Cockayne's syndrome
- Dubowitz syndrome
- Laurence–Moon–Bardet–Biedl syndrome
- Seckel syndrome
- Sjögren–Larsson syndrome
- Smith–Lemli–Opitz syndrome.

X-LINKED RECESSIVE DISORDERS

- Fragile X syndrome
- Lesch–Nyhan syndrome
- Hunter syndrome
- Cerebellar ataxia
- Oculocerebrorenal syndrome (Lowe's syndrome)
- Menke's syndrome.

X-LINKED DOMINANT DISORDERS

- Rett syndrome
- Vitamin D-resistant rickets.

AUTOSOMAL DOMINANT DISORDERS

Tuberose sclerosis (epiloia, Bourneville's disease)
Overall incidence 1:40 000 live births. Autosomal dominant.

Stigmata:

- butterfly rash: begins in crease between cheeks and nose at very young age (angiofibromas)
- '*ade*noma sebaceum'
- *de*ficiency (mental retardation)
- *e*pilepsy
- *shagre*en patches – flesh-coloured, lumbo-sacral plaque-like tumours
- *h*amartomas in lungs and kidneys
- *a*melanotic naevi – macular patches of hypopigmentation (best seen with Wood's light)
- *g*liomas
- *re*tinal phakomas.

Die usually because of heart failure or pneumonia.

Sturge–Weber syndrome (encephalofacial angiomatosis)
50 per cent have mental retardation.
   Epilepsy is common.
   Intracranial angioma (parieto-occipital) – often becomes calcified.
   Cutaneous naevus in distribution of trigeminal nerve (ipsilateral to angioma).

Neurofibromatosis (von Recklinghausen's disease)
Overall incidence 1:3000 live births. A third have mental retardation.
   Stigmata:

- café au lait patches (>5 abnormal)
- pigmentation (melanoma, axillary freckling)
- neural tumours
   - cutaneous neurofibroma, acoustic neuroma, spinal cord nerve root neurofibroma (dumb bell tumour)
   - plexiform neuroma
   - optic nerve glioma
   - meningioma
- aortic coarctation
- berry aneurysm
- obstructive cardiomyopathy
- renal artery stenosis
- diabetes insipidus
- hypospadias
- mesenteric ischaemia
- phaeochromocytoma
- pulmonary fibrosis
- scoliosis
- fibrous dysplasia of bone
- local limb gigantism.

AUTOSOMAL RECESSIVE DISORDERS

Phenylketonuria Folling (1934)

Overall incidence 1:14 000 live births. Third most common known cause of mental retardation (after Down syndrome and Fragile X syndrome).

Absence of phenylalanine hydroxylase. Therefore conversion of phenylalanine (Phe) to tyrosine not possible.

Tested for using the Guthrie test (*B. subtilis* – multiplication phenylalanine dependent). (NB test 6–14 days after birth as levels of amino acid normal at birth.)

Deficiency leads to severe mental retardation (IQ <50). This can be avoided by dietary exclusion of Phe.

Stigmata: ABCDEFGH

- **A**utistic behaviour
- **B**lue eyes
- **C**erebral palsy (visual perception and visual motor skills – more than a third never learn to talk or walk)
- o**D**our (characteristically mousy)
- **E**czema
- **F**its
- **G**rowth is diminished
- **H**air fair (pigmentation deficient).

Tay–Sachs disease (cerebromacular degeneration; amaurotic family idiocy)

Autosomal recessive in children.

- Defect of hexosaminidase A – leads to gradual accumulation of **g**angliosode **G**M2 in **G**rey matter.
- Commonest in **A**shkenazi Jews.
- Earliest sign is hyper-**A**cusis (exaggerated startle).
- T'**AY**'–Sachs: hexosaminidase-**A**.
- Noted sign is macular cherry red spot.

Hurler's disease (gargoylism)

Accumulation of mucopolysaccharidoses in tissues including brain.

Stigmata: THICK

- **TH**ICK long bones
- **H**epatosplenomegaly
- **I**ncrease in head size (disproportionately large)
- **C**orneal clouding
- **K**yphosis.

X-LINKED RECESSIVE DISORDERS

Lesch–Nyan syndrome

Deficiency of hypoxanthine phosphoribosyl transferase in purine metabolism.

Stigmata: LeSCH

- **H**yperuricaemia
- **C**horeoathetosis
- **S**eizures, **S**pasticity, **S**elf-mutilation, **S**mall skull.

Fragile X syndrome (Martin–Bell–Renpenning syndrome)
Overall incidence 1:1000 of general male population.

Second most common known cause of mental retardation in males.

Fragile site (Xq27) – revealed by fragility test (lymphocyte culture in folate-deficient medium).

Stigmata in males:

- perseverative speech which is high pitched and often nasal
- associated with:
  - attention-deficit disorder and autistic disorder (20 per cent of autistics have fragile X syndrome)
  - variable degree of mental retardation
  - short stature
  - flexible joints
  - large ears (floppy)
  - large chin (prognathism)
  - large testicles (macro-orchidism).

Females (1:2000) usually carriers but can express phenotypical features and have mental retardation.

CONDITIONS FEATURING TRINUCLEOTIDE REPEAT

- Fragile X – CGG
- Huntington's disease – CAG
- Myotonic dystrophy – CTG.

X-LINKED DOMINANT DISORDER

Rett's disorder
Progressive degenerative disorder affecting solely females.

Development is normal for first six months of life.

Then manifest:

Hand **S**tereotypies (loss of purposeful movements)	**S**eizures (75 per cent)
Hand wringing	**S**coliosis
Head growth halts or slows down	**S**pasticity
	Small feet
Haphazard movements gait and trunk (ataxia)	**S**peech deficits (receptive/expressive language)
Hyperventilation	**S**ocial interaction/engagement is lost

Neuroimaging

16

Neuroimaging has provided new insights into brain structure and function. In psychiatry the illnesses that have been investigated include schizophrenia, depression, dementia and psychopathy.

Imaging is broadly divided into structural and functional technologies; however, increasingly this separation is becoming less clear.

STRUCTURAL NEUROIMAGING

SKULL RADIOGRAPHY

Using X-rays, the bones of the skull can be visualized. It remains useful in detecting bone pathology and trauma but has been largely superseded by computerized tomography (CT). It is most often used in emergency departments as a screening measure following head injury.

COMPUTERIZED TOMOGRAPHY (CT)

CT images are dependent upon the attenuation, i.e. the loss of energy and slowing, of X-ray photons as they pass through tissues of varying density. Having passed through tissue the emerging X-ray beams are detected and recorded using scintillation counters and, from these data, computer images are mathematically reconstructed and displayed as radiodensity maps. High-density matter, such as bone, appears white and low-density matter, e.g. cerebrospinal fluid, appears black. The CT scan image can be enhanced with the aid of contrast media.

MAGNETIC RESONANCE IMAGING (MRI)

The application of a strong magnetic field aligns the atomic spin axes and produces precession (axial rotation specific to each atom). The delivery of a radiofrequency impulse imparting energy promotes a shift of some nuclei to a higher quantum level (resonance). Subsequent return to their previous level (relaxation) results in the emission of radiofrequency waves that are detected as the magnetic resonance signal. Tissue relaxation is described as T_1 (longitudinal plane – one) and T_2 (transverse plane – two). Alteration of the radiofrequency impulses allows T_1/T_2 weighting, permitting modulation of image specificity. This then allows the derivation of functional information in addition to high resolution structural data.

FUNCTIONAL NEUROIMAGING

SINGLE PHOTON EMISSION COMPUTED TOMOGRAPHY (SPECT/SPET)

A ligand or compound labelled radioactively with an isotope that emits γ photons (radiolabelled ligand/radioisotope) is administered by inhalation, ingestion or intravenous injection. The ligand or compound is chosen on the basis of its specificity for receptors or chemical processes. Its activity can be monitored by computer analysis of its γ photon emissions. From these data images can be constructed called SPECT/SPET scans. Various ligands are used to study receptor density and several compounds are used to examine regional cerebral blood flow (rCBF).

POSITRON EMISSION TOMOGRAPHY (PET)

PET relies on very short-acting radioactive isotopes (e.g. F^{18}, N^{13}, C^{11}) which require on-site synthesis in a **cyclotron**. The positrons that these isotopes emit collide with electrons to produce two γ photons travelling in diametrically opposite directions. These are then detected and recorded, providing data for computer processing from which an image (PET scan) is constructed. PET is more expensive than SPECT but provides images of much greater resolution.

FUNCTIONAL MRI (fMRI)

MRI manipulation can be used to derive functional information (see above). fMRI uses the non-invasive blood oxygenation level-dependent (BOLD) technique to map cortical activation.

MAGNETIC ENCEPHALOGRAPHY (MEG)

MEG is a non-invasive technique that characterizes per millisecond brain electrophysiology by analysing cerebral biomagnetic fields. It can be combined with structural MRI and is useful for:

* localizing epileptiform activity
* mapping of sensorimotor cortex prior to neurosurgery
* characterizing spontaneous abnormal rhythms associated with various neuropathologies.

MAGNETIC RESONANCE SPECTROSCOPY (MRS)

In principle, MRS is similar to structural MRI; however, its focus on chemical composition enables the detection of various metabolites. The most common form of MRS is proton-MRS, which detects metabolites such as *N*-actyl-aspartate (NAA), choline and myo-inositol.

DIFFUSION TENSOR IMAGING (DTI)

This relatively new technique identifies anisotropic diffusion (in white matter) and allows the mapping of tracts. Like spectroscopy this bridges the structural–functional divide.

SIGNIFICANT PSYCHIATRIC NEUROIMAGING FINDINGS

SCHIZOPHRENIA

- *Structural*: CT and MRI
  - non-progressive lateral and third ventricular enlargement
  - reduction in size of superior temporal gyrus, medial temporal lobe and frontal lobe
  - structural abnormalities have been noted in several regions of the brain: hippocampus, parahippocampal gyrus, amygdala and planum temporale
  - thalamic changes implicated in the pathogenesis of schizophrenia
- *Functional*: PET; SECT; fMRI; MRS and MEG
  - hypofrontality (NB some studies have shown ↑ rCBF to L hemisphere and L globus pallidus)
  - auditory hallucinations – localized using fMRI to temporal cortex
  - liddle's symptom clusters:
      psychomotor poverty; ↓ rCBF in L and medial prefrontal cortex disorganization; ↓ rCBF in Broca's area and ↑ perfusion of R medial prefrontal cortex reality distortion; ↑ rCBF in left hippocampal formation
      ↑ response to sensory stimulation
      ↑ response of frontal cortex while performing cognitive tasks
      ↑ synthesis ↑ turnover of dorsolateral prefrontal cortex membrane phospholipids.

AFFECTIVE DISORDERS

- *Structural*
  - ↓ volume of frontal cortex, brainstem, caudate and vermis
  - ↑ ventricular size (inconsistent?) related to cognitive changes and atrophy
  - deep white matter hyperintensities in elderly depressives (especially with late onset: relationship with ischaemic vascular disease) and possibly those with bipolar disorder (associated with poor response to treatment)
  - hippocampal atrophy (especially bipolar disorder)

- amygdala volume loss/enlargement – Bipolar disorder
- pituitary hypertrophy
- adrenal gland hypertrophy
- *Functional*
  - *Depression*
    reversible hypofrontality
    ↓ cingulate cortex rCBF in depressed state. Normalizes with clinical recovery
    limbic-cortical dysregulation model suggests that hypometabolism in dorsal
      brain structures leads to symptoms of psychomotor slowing, apathy and
      attention deficits, whereas hypermetabolism in ventral regions leads to
      disturbed libido, sleep and appetite
    anterior cingulate, orbitofrontal and medial prefrontal cortex and amygdala
      are important in emotion regulation
  - *Bipolar disorder*
    findings are different from those of unipolar depression with possible
      trait and state changes.

DEMENTIA

- *Structural*
  - marked progressive ventricular enlargement is noted in Alzheimer's disease
  - the degree of generalized cortical atrophy and pattern of localized atrophy varies
    according to aetiology
- *Functional*
  - ↓ rCBF, particularly in temporal regions
  - ↑ phosphomonoesterases in Alzheimer's disease
  - proton-MRS has shown decreases of NAA in patients with AD (possible pre-
    clinical marker).

PSYCHOPATHY

- *Structural*
  - ? reduced prefrontal grey matter volume in antisocial personality disorder
- *Functional*
  - prefrontal and limbic regions involved in emotional and learning processes have
    been most often implicated (prefrontal cortex, amygdala and hippocampus).

ANXIETY DISORDERS

- *Structural*
  - ↓ size of R hippocampus in PTSD
- *Functional*
  - ↓ rCBF R parahippocampus in panic disorder
  - ↓ benzodiazepine receptor density in several brain regions of anxious patients.

OBSESSIVE–COMPULSIVE DISORDER (OCD)

- *Structural*
  - ↓ and ↑ of caudate nucleus volume have been noted
- *Functional*
  - caudate nucleus and orbitofrontal cortex changes in metabolism and rCBF
  - rCBF changes normalize with clinical improvement.

ALCOHOLISM

- *Structural*
  - cerebral and cerebellar cortical atrophy
  - extent of cortical atrophy correlates with degree of cognitive impairment
- *Functional*
  - ↓ rCBF (non-specific) correlates with severity of alcohol abuse.

PEPTIDERGIC NEUROTRANSMISSION

Peptides consist of two or more amino acids joined by **peptide bonds**. They are smaller than proteins with a molecular weight less than 10 kDa. Their structure is described left to right from the N-terminus (end with an amino group) to the C-terminus (end with carboxyl group). Neuropeptides are synthesized as prepropeptides. These possess an N-terminus signal sequence consisting of hydrophobic amino acids. The signal sequence ('pre' portion of prepropeptide) facilitates entry of the prepropeptide into endoplasmic reticulum where it is cleaved to form a propeptide. This is then chemically modified prior to secretion.

Catabolism of peptides is carried out by specific peptides that are important in terminating their neurotransmitter functions.

Neuropeptides (peptide transmitters) differ from classic transmitters in several important ways (see Table 17.1).

CO-LOCALIZATION (COEXISTENCE) OF TRANSMITTERS

Sir John Eccles formalized Dale's principle stating that the different terminals of a particular neurone/cell should behave in a similar fashion and thereby release the same

Table 17.1 Classic and peptide neurotransmitters

	Classic neurotransmitter	Peptide neurotransmitter
Precursor synthesis	No	Yes (prepropeptide).
Converting enzymes	No	Yes
Synthesized in soma	No (not usually)	Yes
Synthesized in terminals	Yes	No (not usually)
Effective concentrations	Micromolar/nanomolar	Picomolar
Relative rate of synthesis	Fast	Slow
Receptor affinity	High	Low
Receptor potency	Low	High
Neuronal re-uptake	Yes	No (not significant)

Table 17.2 Neurotransmitter co-localization

Neurotransmitter	Co-localized neuropeptide	Neurones
Acetylcholine	Vasoactive intestinal peptide	Cortical and parasympathetic
Dopamine	Cholecystokinin	Ventrotegmental
Noradrenaline	Neuropeptide Y	Brainstem
Gamma-aminobutyric acid GABA	Somatostatin	Hippocampal
Serotonin	Thyroid-releasing hormone (TRH) and Substance P	Medulla

transmitter. The assertion is that neurones display chemical unity/uniformity, and the principle does not address the number of transmitters a neurone/cell uses.

Transmitter co-localization is a relatively recent discovery which adds to the complexity of neurotransmission. Co-localized transmitters may act as **neuromodulators**. That is, they modulate the action of a co-existent transmitter rather than effecting actions themselves. This may be achieved by interacting with the transmitter directly or through receptors on the same or different neurones.

Table 17.2 gives examples that have been shown to co-exist.

CLASSIFICATION

Neuropeptides can be grouped as follows:

1 **Hypothalamic releasing hormones**
   - corticotrophin-releasing factor (CRF)
   - thyrotrophin-releasing hormone (TRH)
   - somatostatin
   - gonadotrophin-releasing hormone
   - growth hormone-releasing hormone (GHRH)
2 **Pituitary hormones**
   - oxytocin ⎫
   - vasopressin ⎭ (posterior pituitary)
   - adrenocorticotrophic hormone (ACTH)
   - thyroid-stimulating hormone (TSH) ⎫ from basophils
   - luteinizing hormone (LH)
   - follicle-stimulating hormone (FSH)
   - growth hormone (GH) ⎫ from acidophils
   - prolactin (PRL) ⎭
3 **Gut-brain peptides**
   - vasoactive intestinal peptide (VIP)
   - cholecystokinin (CCK)
   - substance P
   - neuropeptide Y
   - neurotensin
   - insulin
   - glucagon

4 **Opioid peptides**
   – leu-enkephalin
   – met-enkephalin
   – β-endorphin
   – dynorphin
5 **Others**
   – calcitonin-gene-related peptide (CGRP)
   – bradykinin
   – orexins.

ENDOGENOUS OPIOID PEPTIDES

These fall into three groups derived from separate precursor polypeptides:

Enkephalins: derived from proenkephalins. Are widely distributed throughout central and peripheral nervous systems. Met-enkephalin and leu-enkephalin are pentapeptides.

Endorphins: derived from pro-opiomelanocortin (POMC) in pituitary anterior and intermediate lobes and hypothalamic arcuate nucleus. POMC gives rise to β-endorphin and also contains amino acid sequences for β-lipotropin, ACTH and melanocyte-stimulating hormone.

Dynorphins: derived from prodynorphin.

There are three main classes of central nervous system opioid receptors: μ (mu), κ (kappa) and δ (delta). These are concentrated in hypothalamic, limbic and sensory brain regions and in particular the amygdala and periaqueductal grey matter.

The G-protein-coupled opioid receptors inhibit neurotransmission by diminishing the release of other neurotransmitters (DA, ACh, 5-HT).

κ receptors are calcium-channel linked (decrease Ca^{2+} entry), as may be μ and δ receptors in certain tissues.

μ receptors and δ receptors are also potassium-channel linked (increase K^+ conductance), and all three types of receptor can inhibit adenylate cyclase.

Endogenous opioids are involved in addiction, dependence, analgesia, learning and memory, and opioid receptor changes have been implicated in affective disorders and schizophrenia.

VASOACTIVE INTESTINAL PEPTIDE (VIP)

Found in autonomic ganglia, intestinal and respiratory tracts and in the cerebral cortex, hypothalamus, amygdala and hippocampus. VIP stimulates the release of ACTH, growth hormone and prolactin and inhibits the release of somatostatin. It also produces neuronal excitation.

SOMATOSTATIN

Plays an important role in inhibiting the release of growth hormone and generally has inhibitory effects. It is concentrated in the cerebral cortex and limbic system and is diminished in dementia (Alzheimer's disease). It has an excitatory effect on hippocampal pyramidal cells.

CHOLECYSTOKININ (CCK)

CCK-8 is the most prevalent of its three forms (CCK-33 and CCK-39) and is found especially in the amygdala, hippocampus and cerebral cortex, where it has excitatory effects. It is thought to act on dopamine pathways and is important in mechanisms of satiety, analgesia, panic and anxiety.

NEUROTENSIN

Co-existence with DA and modulation of DA-related behaviour. Putative target for treatment of schizophrenia.

SUBSTANCE P AND NEUROKININS A AND B

Receptors NK_{1-3}: possible targets for antipsychotics and antidepressants.

OREXINS

Hypocretins (orexins A and B) are derived from a single gene. They are involved in stress and circadian functions and act on OX_1 and OX_2 receptors found in the lateral hypothalamus.

NEUROENDOCRINOLOGY

Specialized hypothalamic cells release neuropeptides that act on anterior pituitary cells to release peptide hormones. These then enter the systemic circulation and are able to act on specific organs/tissues (Figures 17.1 and 17.2).

There are several neuroendocrine axes that function in this manner: they are usually described with particular reference to the end-organ, e.g. the adrenal and thyroid axes, or the specific hormone of interest, e.g. the growth hormone and the gonadotrophin axes.

These neuropeptides and the end-organ hormones exert negative-feedback control. The release of the hypothalamic neuropeptides is also influenced by neurotransmitters.

Neuroendocrine studies have revealed significant changes in several psychiatric disorders.

HPA AXIS (see Figure 17.3)

CRF from the hypothalamic paraventricular nucleus (PVN) travels in the hypothalamic-hypophysealportal-system to the anterior pituitary where it acts to yield ACTH

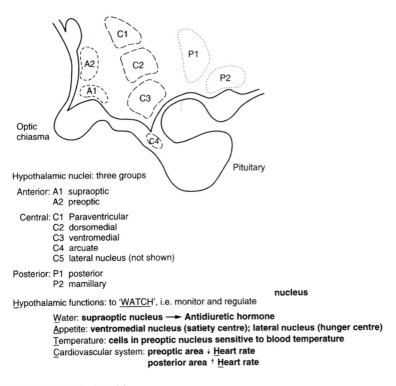

Optic
chiasma

Pituitary

Hypothalamic nuclei: three groups

Anterior: A1 supraoptic
         A2 preoptic

Central: C1 Paraventricular
         C2 dorsomedial
         C3 ventromedial
         C4 arcuate
         C5 lateral nucleus (not shown)

Posterior: P1 posterior
           P2 mamillary

Hypothalamic functions: to 'WATCH', i.e. monitor and regulate

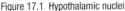

         Water: **supraoptic nucleus** ⟶ **Antidiuretic hormone**
         Appetite: **ventromedial nucleus (satiety centre); lateral nucleus (hunger centre)**
         Temperature: **cells in preoptic nucleus sensitive to blood temperature**
         Cardiovascular system: **preoptic area ↓ Heart rate**
                                posterior area ↑ Heart rate

Figure 17.1 Hypothalamic nuclei

from POMC. ACTH released into the bloodstream acts on the adrenal cortex resulting in the release of cortisol (see Figure 17.3).

CRF receptor (CRF_1 and CRF_2) antagonists are being evaluated as potential antidepressants.

The brain possesses two types of 'steroid receptor':

- *mineralocorticoid receptors (type I)* have a high affinity for cortisol and are to be found mainly in the septo-hippocampal complex
- *glucocorticoid receptors (type II)* have less affinity for cortisol and are more widely distributed.

Both types of receptor participate in HPA-axis negative feedback. Negative feedback has been shown to be fast, intermediate and slow. Slow feedback occurs over a period of hours and involves the inhibition of pituitary ACTH synthesis. Intermediate feedback occurs over a period of minutes. It is concentration dependent and diminishes ACTH secretion. Fast feedback is rate sensitive and inhibits ACTH secretion in a matter of seconds following a rapid increase of plasma cortisol.

Normally the HPA axis has a circadian rhythm. Peak cortisol secretion occurs early morning and it falls to its lowest late evening.

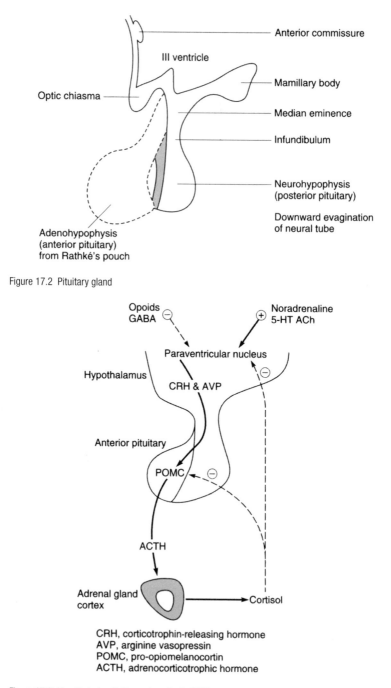

Figure 17.2 Pituitary gland

Figure 17.3 Hypothalmic-pituitary-adrenal axis (HPA)

HPA ABNORMALITIES

DEPRESSION

- Cortisol hypersecretion (50 per cent of patients) with increased urinary excretion (2× normal)
- Adrenal gland volume shows 70 per cent ↑ (magnetic resonance imaging (MRI))
- Pituitary gland enlargement
- ↑ CSF CRH (depressed patients and suicides)
- ↓ CRH receptor-binding sites in frontal cortex of suicides
- Dexamethasone suppression test non-suppression (50–70 per cent of major depressives; >90 per cent of those with psychotic depression)*
- Blunted ACTH/cortisol responses to CRH
- Blunted ACTH/cortisol responses to ipsapirone (5-HT$_{1A}$ agonist)
- HPA abnormalities (particularly hypercortisolaemia and DST non-suppression) usually normalize with clinical recovery.

*not specific, also found in: OCD; dementia; panic disorder; eating disorders; alcohol withdrawal; normal population (5–10 per cent).

SCHIZOPHRENIA

- Normal ACTH/cortisol response to CRH
- Dexamethasone non-suppression may occur in acute episodes of schizophrenia (contentious findings), however, it has rarely been observed in patients with chronic schizophrenia.

ALZHEIMER'S DISEASE

- Hypercortisolaemia
- Dexamethasone non-suppression (>50 per cent of patients).

THYROID AXIS ABNORMALITIES

Hypothalamic TRH travels in the hypophyseal portal system to the anterior pituitary gland where it stimulates the synthesis and release of TSH. TSH releases the thyroid hormones tri-iodothyronine (T$_3$) and thyroxine (T$_4$) from the thyroid gland. Axis function is influenced by TSH and thyroid hormone negative feedback, and is inhibited by somatostatin.

DEPRESSION

- ↑ TSH levels (subclinical hypothyroidism) especially common in those with bipolar affective disorder
- Blunted response to TRH stimulation in about 30 per cent of depressives; this remains despite clinical recovery in about 15 per cent and seems to be associated with increased likelihood of relapse
- ↑ CSF TRH levels

- 20 per cent have anti-thyroid antibodies (more than twice the level in normal population).

PROLACTIN AXIS ABNORMALITIES

PRL is released from anterior pituitary cells in response to TRH, AVP and VIP. Dopamine inhibits the release of PRL whereas serotonin and its amino-acid precursor tryptophan enhance its release (indirectly).

DEPRESSION

PRL release is blunted in response to:

- tryptophan
- D-fenfluramine (causes 5-HT release and inhibits its re-uptake)
- clomipramine.

GROWTH HORMONE AXIS ABNORMALITIES

Pituitary GH release is stimulated by GHRH and inhibited by somatostatin. The release of these neuropeptides is influenced by neurotransmitters ACh, DA and NA (Figure 17.4).

GH is released in pulses and peaks with the onset of slow-wave sleep. Its release is stimulated by stress, hypoglycaemia, exercise, sleep, surgery and pyrexia, and inhibited by negative feedback.

DEPRESSION

- GH release is blunted in response to:
  - hypoglycaemia (insulin tolerance test)
  - **clonidine** (α_2-agonist)
  - **desipramine**
- GH release increased in response to **pyridostigmine** (anticholinesterase)
- Reduced nocturnal secretion
- ↓ CSF somatostatin.

SCHIZOPHRENIA AND ALZHEIMER'S DISEASE (TENTATIVE FINDING)

- ↓ CSF somatostatin

NEUROENDOCRINE ABNORMALITIES IN EATING DISORDERS AND OCD

ANOREXIA NERVOSA

- ↓ plasma T_3 (NB T_4 level normal)
- ↓ plasma oestrogen and gonadotrophins.

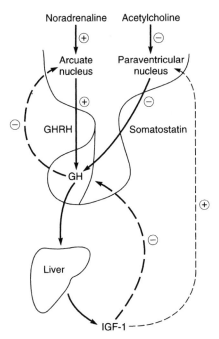

GH, growth hormone
GHRH, growth hormone-releasing hormone
IGF-1, insulin-like growth factor

Figure 17.4 Growth hormone axis

ANOREXIA NERVOSA AND BULIMIA NERVOSA

- ↑ plasma GH
- ↑ plasma cortisol
- ↑ plasma cholecystokinin (CCK)
- Dexamethasone non-suppression.

OBSESSIVE–COMPULSIVE DISORDER (OCD)

- Blunted prolactin and cortisol responses to D-**fenfluramine** challenge
- Normal responses to clonidine and **desipramine** challenge
- Normal dexamethasone suppression
- Enhanced GH response to pyridostigmine.

Statistics

Statistics is the collection and interpretation of observations, a method for translating **data** (numerical information) into something we can understand. A **statistic** can mean various things, but in the context of this chapter it is any piece of information gleaned from the primary data.

As with any interpretative process, conclusions drawn from research data may lie anywhere on a spectrum of accuracy. Assessing the quality of a research paper, by considering the integrity of the original observations and how they have been interpreted, is the remit of **critical appraisal**:

1 **What was done?** – There should be a clear statement both of intent and of an end point, so the reader can decide whether the paper is of interest to them and whether the investigators actually completed what they set out to do in the manner they specified.
2 **Who did it?** – Helps identify possible conflicts of interest and whether the investigators were qualified to conduct the research.
3 **Why did they do it?** – What does the paper add to the existing knowledge base and why is this important?
4 **How was it done?** – What methods were used to collect the data and then extract the information from it? How well were these methods executed?

Critical appraisal is usually undertaken by **peer review**; a group of people deemed to have sufficient expertise in research techniques and the subject matter put the paper through a check-list such as the one above. An individual clinician may further ask:

5 **Can I use it?** – Is it possible to implement the results or recommendations in my own clinical setting?

A **variable** is something that can change and so requires measuring each time we want to know what it is. Variables can be fixed relative to one another. For example, if we measure the height of a group of 6 year olds, age is invariant (i.e. fixed) and height is the variable. On the other hand, if we measure the ages of a group of people 3 feet tall, height is invariant and age is now the variable.

Medical research is generally concerned with looking for differences between groups, but the cause of any potential difference can be lost among the multiple variables present in any group of people. Usually, as many variables as possible are fixed (**matched/controlled**) between groups, with the exception of the one the investigators are interested in measuring.

A **parametric** variable is one that follows a mathematical rule (i.e. repeated measurements of the variable build up a pattern or graph of some kind); non-parametric variables do not.

Independent variables are those that are fixed or manipulated directly by the investigator, and **dependent** variables are those that change as a result (i.e. they are influenced by the independent variables). If it is not clear which is which, it is generally safe to assume that the dependent variable is the one the investigators are interested in.

Quantitative information can be measured and expressed as a number; an individual measurement generates a unit of data. It can be categorized using interval and ratio scales (see Chapter 4) and is either **discrete** (limited to a finite number of possibilities) or **continuous** (not limited). Note that continuous data may be restricted to a particular range but not to a particular number of values. For example, we can be certain that a piece of string cut from a spool 1 m long will be between 0 and 1 m, but there is no theoretical limit to the number of places along the string we might make the cut.

Qualitative information cannot be reduced to numbers and so requires different analytical techniques from quantitative information. It is categorized using nominal or ordinal scales.

A **population** is the group under study (a 'population' might be anything, not just people). It is usually too large to be considered in its entirety and so is sampled to provide a more manageable number of subjects. A good **sample** is thus a representative proportion of the population, i.e. its attributes accurately reflect those of the population from which it has been derived.

A **parameter** is a particular attribute of some aspect of a population, e.g. the mean age or the standard deviation of the heights. Since these values cannot be known for certain without measuring the entire population, they are instead approximated by the sample statistics. That is, the sample statistics (e.g. mean $\bar{x}$, standard deviation s, correlation r) are estimates of population parameters (μ, σ and ρ respectively).

An **arm** (or limb) of a study is a particular path or protocol followed by a subdivision of the sample. Different arms are therefore different pathways, along which subjects will be treated differently.

An **audit** measures what *should* happen. Note that this implies a pre-established standard (i.e. one that is not re-evaluated or measured during the course of the audit) against which the data are then compared. Research aims to measure what *actually* happens, and may (where applicable) assess whether the data fit with a particular hypothesis.

PRIMARY RESEARCH

Collects and analyses novel/original information.

Observational: descriptive without attempting to create a systematic difference (though the purpose is often to look for one).

- *Case–control*: individuals with a particular condition (cases) are matched with individuals without the condition (controls). Both groups' histories are then trawled for a significant difference in some putative aetiological factor. Useful for investigating rare conditions or those with a long latency.

- *Cohort*: individuals with a particular attribute/exposure are matched to individuals without. Both groups are then monitored forward in time for the development of a pre-determined outcome (typically a disease).
- *Survey*: the collection and interpretation of data without undertaking a systematic intervention. *Cross-sectional* if done once, *longitudinal* if repeated at least once (cohort studies are essentially longitudinal surveys of two or more groups conducted in parallel).
- *Case report*: a single-patient episode/history deemed to be of interest or educational value.
- *n of 1*: study involving a single subject.

Experimental: attempts to prove a systematic difference through making a specific intervention.

- *Randomized Controlled Trial (RCT)*: individuals are randomly given or spared a specific intervention (the other variables having been controlled for), then compared after a pre-determined time for a significant difference in some pre-specified measure.
- *Pragmatic*: similar to an RCT but conducted without matching in an effort to better simulate real life and avoid the criticism of 'diagnostic purity'.
- *Non-randomized controlled*: similar to an RCT but without randomization; necessary in situations where randomization is unethical or unachievable. Particular care should be taken to specify the initial differences between the groups, as well as the differences at the end.
- *Cross-over*: sample is not split into different groups, but is instead given each of the interventions one after the other, 'crossing over' at a pre-determined time; subjects act as their own controls. Correctly matching the right effect to the right intervention, and possible interference between them, can be problematic. However, such studies can be useful in studying rare disorders, where only a limited number of subjects may be available.
- *Open*: all subjects are given the same treatment (i.e. there are no controls).

SECONDARY RESEARCH

Collects and analyses primary research.

- *Review*: a survey of the published literature on a topic. May be systematic/non-systematic.
- *Meta-analysis*: takes a number of similarly conducted research papers on a particular topic (typically RCTs) and combines their results.
- *Economic analysis*: measures the costs/benefits (not necessarily just monetary) of clinical practices to help inform decisions about resource allocation.
- *Guidelines*: suggested protocols based on 'best available evidence', which may include reviews/meta-analyses/RCTs/economic analyses etc.

HIERARCHY OF EVIDENCE

Papers are weighted for apparent scientific rigor according to the following convention adopted by the National Institute for Clinical Excellence (NICE):

1 Meta-analysis of RCTs
2 At least 1 RCT
3 At least 1 non-randomized controlled trial
4 Other experimental studies
5 Other semi-experimental studies
6 Descriptive studies (e.g. case–control, cohort)
7 Opinion (committee > expert > anecdotal)

DATA COLLECTION

The fundamental question to consider is 'what are the potential differences between information gleaned from the sample and that which might be gleaned from the population (other than those **deliberately** produced by the study), and how can these be minimized?'.

Bias: anything that influences the **collection** of data, causing them to be under/over-estimated or recorded. There are many potential kinds and sources of bias, but the main ones occur in sample recruitment and information gathering. In either case, bias can be introduced by the subjects or the investigators and can be positive or negative. *Examples* are:

- *Sampling bias*: a non-representative proportion of the population is identified and/or recruited by the study. Consider how and from where the sample was recruited: was everyone in the target population equally likely to have been chosen? Strictly, inclusion/exclusion criteria and the matching process render a sample unrepresentative, which is an argument for pragmatic trials
- *Response bias*: a non-representative proportion of the population agrees to partake in the study (only relevant if the sample was correctly identified in the first place)
- *Interviewer bias*: investigator's objectivity is compromised by their perception of the subject or the subject's group status
- *Hawthorne effect*: subject's objectivity is compromised by the fact that they know they are being studied
- *Halo effect*: subject or investigator tries to make the data 'fit'
- *Recall bias*: e.g. mothers of children with learning difficulties are more likely to recall possible causative factors than controls are (i.e. mothers with healthy children).

Counter-measures:

- *Randomization*: in sampling – all members of the target population have an equal chance of being recruited into the sample; in RCTs – all recruits have an equal chance of being subjects or controls
- *Concealment*: the randomization is kept secret from the subjects and investigators

- *Blinding/masking*: being unaware of the subject's group status. Single – subjects are unaware; double – subjects and investigators are unaware; triple – subjects, investigators and an independent group who analyse the results are all unaware
- *Standardized assessment*: minimizes the potential for interviewer bias
- *Guessing*: blind investigators record which group they think subjects belong to and later compare these guesses against the subjects' true status in order to estimate the degree of potential there may have been for interviewer bias.

Confounding: anything that influences the **manifestation** of data, causing it be under/over-estimated or recorded. Confounders are not directly causative or curative; instead, they interact with the observation of interest (attribute/outcome/disease etc.) in a systematic way to produce a consistent deviation in **how** and to **what degree** it is expressed.
Counter-measures:

- *Matching*: confounders are 'matched' between groups so they will essentially cancel each other out. Common examples are age and sex
- *Restriction*: optimizing the inclusion/exclusion criteria to minimize known confounders
- *Statistical control*: if it is possible to estimate the size of the deviation, it can be partially compensated for in the calculations.

DATA DESCRIPTION

Once we are confident the data are accurate and valid, we can move on to interpreting what they mean. It must be established what kind of data they are (qualitative/quantitative, discrete/continuous etc.) as this will determine the most appropriate method of analysis.

The first stage of data analysis is to describe them. The authors of any paper should therefore strive for both clarity and completeness in presenting their data, by giving as much information as possible (e.g. sample number, demographics, breakdown of subjects vs. controls etc.) and making sure the 'numbers add up'.

Everyone who entered the study should have been accounted for by the end, and the reader left in no doubt as to what the data represent. This is often a good way to start the analysis, and helps to build up a picture of what actually happened to subjects during the course of the study.

There is generally no right or wrong way of displaying data, though some may be more appropriate than others depending on the type of data, how much data there is and what the authors are trying to demonstrate. Often, a simple visual inspection of a good display will yield useful information about trends and relationships within the data.

- *Box-whisker plot*: the box spans the inter-quartile range (see below) and the 'whiskers' (vertical lines) span down from the 1st and up from the 3rd quartile to the lowest and highest value respectively. The median is sometimes marked within the box. Useful for large data sets, where it is not practical to plot individual data points. However, *n* (the size of the sample) should still be stated.
- *Bar chart*: a frequency display used for discrete variables. The height of the bars represents the frequency of a particular category of variable.

- *Histogram*: a frequency display for continuous variables. There should be no gaps between the boxes (because there are no gaps in a continuous variable). The frequency pattern is easier to discern with equal-width bars. Look out for overlap, e.g. 0–1, 1–2, 2–3, 3–4 etc.
- *Scattergram*: useful for plotting individual data points.

Other examples of data displays are tables, graphs, pie charts (only show relative proportions) etc. Particular attention should always be paid to the legend, labelling and scales used in visual displays.

When rounding numbers, **significant figures** are the number of digits to be included from left to right, the rest being replaced by 0. For example, 1235 and 1.235 rounded to 2 significant figures are 1200 and 1.2 respectively. Rounding to a certain number of **decimal places** is the same procedure but applied to numbers occurring after a decimal point. For example, 1235 and 1.235 rounded to 2 decimal places are 1235 and 1.24 respectively (if the first digit to be rounded is $\geqslant 5$ the preceding digit is increased by 1, so in this case the 3 becomes a 4). When answering statistical questions, it is good practice to use the same system of rounding as used in the data or question.

Occasionally researchers may **transform** their data in order to make them easier to work with. A common example is to take the logarithm, which can sometimes convert skewed data into a normal distribution (see below) and so allow parametric tests to be carried out (parametric tests are more robust than non-parametric ones). The log of a number is the power to which the base must be raised to give that number (i.e. if $\log_{10} x = y$, then $10^y = x$). Common bases are 10 (log) and e (ln), a naturally occurring constant like π. It is important to keep track of whether the data are in their original or transformed state.

USEFUL SYMBOLS

- n: the size of a sample
- N: size of the population
- x: a numerical variable
- Σ: 'sum of', e.g. $\Sigma(1, 3, 7, 2, 4, 6) = 23$. Where Σ is used with a variable, it means 'sum of all the values represented by that variable', e.g. Σx = sum of (all values of x), $\Sigma(x - \bar{x})$ = sum of (x minus the mean of x) for all values of x (note that in this example $\bar{x}$ represents a fixed number which does not have different values).
- $\bar{x}$: sample mean
- μ: population mean
- s: sample standard deviation (also s.d. or S.D.)
- σ: population standard deviation

MEASURES OF CENTRAL TENDENCY

The value 'most representative' of the data:

- *Mean*: sum of all the values divided by the number of values. Restricted to interval and ratio variables (Table 18.1). Can be distorted by extreme values (e.g. mean of 1, 6, 3, 6, 4, 100 is 20).

Table 18.1 Types of scales to which measures of central tendency can be applied

Measure	Scale			
	Nominal	Ordinal	Interval	Ratio
Mean			+	+
Median		+	+	+
Mode	+	+	+	+

- *Median*: the middle value when ranked in order. With an even number of values, the median is given by the mean of the middle two (e.g. median of 1, 3, 4, 6, 6, 100 is 5). The median is less sensitive to extreme values than the mean and can also be used with ordinal scales.
- *Mode*: the most common value within a distribution, i.e. that occurring most frequently (e.g. in the above example it is 6). There may be more than one mode if more than one value occurs equally frequently or has the same probability. The mode can be used for data measured on a nominal scale.

MEASURES OF DISPERSION

How 'spread out' the data are:

- *Range*: determined by the highest and lowest values. It is distorted by extreme values and can be applied only to values measured on an interval or ratio scale. It may be stated as a single number (highest – lowest) or two numbers (lowest, highest)
- *Quantiles*: these are individual ranges of data created by 'splitting' the original data at the median value over and again (i.e. the data are split half-way, then the two halves are each split at the half-way point again, and so on), so that each quantile contains the same number of values (but not necessarily the same range of values).
  Hence, if the data are split into 4 (i.e. 'quartiles'), 25 per cent of the data lie beneath Q1, 50 per cent beneath Q2 (the median), 75 per cent beneath Q3 and 100 per cent beneath Q4. The inter-quartile range (IQR) is a measure of dispersion and spans the 1st quartile to the 3rd (i.e. from 25 per cent to 75 per cent of the data). The semi-IQR is the IQR/2. Similarly, if the data are split into 100 ('centiles' or 'percentiles'), 2 per cent of the data lies beneath the 2nd centile, 50 per cent beneath the 50th centile (the median), 89 per cent beneath the 89th centile and so on
- *Variance*: a measure of the total degree of difference between the values and their mean. The difference between the mean and each value is squared (so the positives do not cancel the negatives) and then added together. The result is then divided by N for a population or $n - 1$ for a sample ($n - 1$ represents the 'degrees of freedom'; the explanation for using this value is beyond the scope of this book):

$$\sigma^2 = \frac{\Sigma(x - \mu)^2}{N}$$

(or a more calculator-friendly: $\sigma^2 = \Sigma x^2/N - \mu^2$)

$$s^2 = \frac{\Sigma(x - \bar{x})^2}{(n - 1)} = \frac{1}{(n - 1)}\left[\Sigma x^2 - \frac{\Sigma(x)^2}{n}\right]$$

(or: $s^2 = n\sigma^2/(n - 1)$)

The closer the values are to the mean, the smaller the variance

- *Standard deviation*: the square root of the variance, and so expressed in the same units as the data.

STANDARD ERROR

Because statistics such as the mean and variance of a sample are only estimates of the true population parameters, they may of course be wrong. The **standard error** (SE) is used to indicate the degree of accuracy of these estimates. As you would expect, the SE depends on the degree of data dispersion. The larger the sample (i.e. the larger the number of subjects included from the population), the smaller the standard error and the more accurate the estimate.

The standard error of a statistic (e.g. sample mean) is in effect a measure of the dispersion of the various estimates we would obtain for that statistic if we were to take multiple samples. It turns out such that estimates (i.e. those based on samples from the same population) follow the normal distribution, which allows us to calculate their confidence limits (see below).

Note that the SE should be used when making estimates or inferences about population parameters from a sample. The standard deviation is simply a measure of data dispersion.

$$\mathrm{SE}\,\bar{x} = s/\sqrt{n}$$

Standard errors can also be calculated for proportions, odds ratios and other sample statistics.

RISK/ODDS/PROBABILITY

Odds are a way of expressing the likelihood of an outcome. They are not the same as probability, though essentially they measure the same thing (just as miles and kilometres are not the same but both measure distance). Risk and probability are the same.

If P is the probability of an event then odds $(O) = P/(1 - P)$. Odds are usually expressed as two numbers; the number of times an event occurs vs. the number of times it does not occur (this order is adopted by convention). So, if the odds of an event are expressed as 2:6 (or '2 to 6' or '2/6' etc.), this means that out of every 8 trials (2 + 6) the event is expected to occur twice. If odds are expressed as a single number, in this case 2/6 (which can be reduced to 1/3), it is important to realize this value is higher than the probability (which is $\frac{1}{4}$, i.e. 1 out of 4).

The *odds ratio* (OR) of a 2 × 2 table is given by the odds of the event in one group divided by the odds of the event in the other group, e.g. the OR of group A to group B in Table 18.2 is given by $(a/b)/(c/d) = (ad/bc)$.

Table 18.2

	Event occurred *or* Positive test result	Event did not occur *or* Negative test result	Total
A [control group] *or* Lack attribute	a b	b	a + b
B [experiment group] *or* Have attribute	c d	d	c + d
	a + c	b + d	

- *Relative risk* (RR): the risk of an event in one group relative to the risk of the event in another group, i.e. the probability of the event occurring in group A divided by the probability of it occurring in group B: $[a/(a + b)]/[c/(c + d)]$. For example, a RR of 0.12 means the event is 0.12 times as likely to occur in group A as in group B (a RR of less than 1 means the event is less likely, more than 1 means it is more likely).

- *Absolute risk reduction* (ARR): the difference in risk (probability) of an event between two groups: $a/(a + b) - c/(c + d)$. For example, an ARR of 0.12 means the probability of the event in group A is 0.12 greater than its probability in group B (the ARR can only lie between 0 and 1).

  Probabilities can never be negative, and so in taking the 'absolute' value (i.e. ignoring the sign) it is important to note which way around the calculation has been done. If the risk is actually increased (in considering the impact of an exposure in a cohort study for example), this difference is termed the **absolute risk increase** (ARI).

- *Relative risk reduction* (RRR): the ARR of an event relative to the actual risk of that event in a group. In Table 18.2, the RRR in the experiment group is given by $ARR/[c/(c + d)]$. When considering an ARI instead, this statistic is termed **relative risk increase**. Unlike absolute risk, the relative risk helps to gain perspective by taking into consideration how large or small the actual risks are.

  For example, if the probability of an event is 0.90 in group A and 0.89 in group B (high baseline risk), the ARR is $(0.9 - 0.89) = 0.01$. If instead the probabilities were 0.02 and 0.01 respectively (low baseline risk), the ARR would still be 0.01 but the RRR of the event in the high baseline group A is only $0.01/0.9 = 0.011$ but $0.01/0.02 = 0.5$ in the low baseline group A; the same reduction has a greater 'impact' in the low baseline group.

- *Number needed to treat* (NNT): 1/ARR (the value is usually rounded up to the nearest whole number). An NNT of 5 means that for every 5 subjects treated in each of the experimental and control groups, 1 extra event will have occurred in the experimental group. It can be seen that the smaller the ARR, the larger the NNT (i.e. the more subjects will have to be treated in order to notice a difference between the groups).

  Depending on the circumstances of the study, different researchers may regard different NNTs as being clinically useful or relevant. If the study is looking at adverse events, or when considering an ARI, the statistic is termed the **number needed to harm** (NNH).

- *Sensitivity* (of a test): proportion of people with the attribute who have a positive result. So, for Table 18.2, the sensitivity is given by $c/(c + d)$. The more sensitive a test, the greater the proportion of people with the attribute who will have a positive result (and so the smaller the proportion of these people who will have a negative result). Hence, if a sensitive test yields a negative result, the likelihood of it being wrong is low.

- *Specificity* (of a test): proportion of people without the attribute who have a negative result. For Table 18.2, this is $b/(a + b)$. The more specific a test, the greater the proportion of people without the attribute who will have a negative result (and so the smaller the proportion of these people who will have a positive result). Hence if a specific test yields a positive result, the likelihood of it being wrong is low.
- *Efficiency (or accuracy)*: proportion of all tests that are correct. For Table 18.2, this is $(c + b)/(a + b + c + d)$.
- *Positive predictive value, PPV* (of a test): the likelihood of actually having the test attribute, given a positive result; i.e. proportion of people who have the disease out of those who tested positive. For Table 18.2, this is $c/(a + c)$.
- *Negative predictive value, NPV* (of a test): the likelihood of not having the attribute, given a negative result; i.e. proportion of people who do not have the disease out of those who tested negative. For Table 18.2, this is given by $b/(b + d)$.
- *Attributable risk*: the difference in the risk of an outcome (e.g. illness) between those exposed and those not exposed to a particular intervention or factor. This statistic may, for example, be quoted in a cohort study when considering the additional (i.e. attributable) risk posed by a particular event or attribute.
- *Likelihood ratio, LR* (of a test): The ratio of how likely a result is to be correct rather than incorrect, i.e. how likely a person with a positive result is to have the attribute than not, and vice versa.
  LR for a positive result = true positives/false positives = c/a. LR for a negative result = true negatives/false negatives = b/d.
- *Pre-test odds*: the prevalence of the test attribute among the target population. The pre-test probability is given by $P = O/(1 + O)$.
- *Post-test odds*: the prevalence of the test attribute among those who have the test. For a positive result, post-test odds = LR(+ve result) × pre-test odds; post-test odds (−ve result) = LR(−ve result) × pre-test odds.

THE NORMAL (OR GAUSSIAN) DISTRIBUTION

Distributions are mathematical 'patterns' created by certain variables. Establishing that a variable conforms to a particular distribution is helpful because it means it follows the rules of that distribution, making available a ready-made bank of assumptions and mathematical techniques (since these have already been worked out).

Many variables in nature and medical literature conform to the normal distribution. This is a particular type of distribution that applies to independent continuous data that is symmetrical about the mean ('bell-shaped'). Calculating individual probabilities in this distribution is difficult and also not that useful, so instead the probability of a range of values is considered (i.e. the probability of a variable being higher or lower than a particular value). The normal distribution can also be used to analyse data from large samples even if the variable itself is not normally distributed.

Because there are many different instances of the normal distribution, with different means and variances, it is useful to convert an individual value from one of these distributions to its equivalent in the so-called 'standard normal distribution'. This is the normal distribution with mean 0 and standard deviation 1. The converted value is called the **z-score**, and denotes the number of standard deviations a value is away from the mean:

$$z = (x - \bar{x})/s$$

Due to the symmetry of the distribution about the mean, we can say that the probability of a value being above a negative z-score is identical to the probability of a value being below the positive value of the same z-score (and vice versa).

The probabilities of the standard normal distribution have been worked out and are available in tables. The probabilities of any normal variable can therefore be obtained by first calculating its z-score and then looking this up in a table. If the probability is required in the opposite direction to that given (different tables may quote the probability above or below the z-score), subtracting from 1 will give the required result (since the summed total of any probability distribution is always 1).

It is also important to note whether the particular table being consulted gives a one-tailed or two-tailed probability, i.e. does it quote the probability on only one side of z (e.g. probability of $z > 1.96$) or on either side of plus and minus z (e.g. probabilities of $z < -1.96$ plus $z > 1.96$).

It turns out that 90 per cent of the values in a normal distribution lie within 1.645 standard deviations on either side of the mean, 95 per cent within 1.96 standard deviations, and 99 per cent within 2.576 standard deviations. In other words, the probability of z lying outside ± 1.645 is 0.1; outside ± 1.96 is 0.05; and outside ± 2.576 is 0.01.

Note that these probabilities relate to a range (and also that these are two-tailed results). The probability of an individual z-score can be calculated by computer and is referred to as the **P-value**.

OTHER DISTRIBUTIONS

A **binomial** probability distribution describes the frequency with which a discrete random event (of fixed probability) occurs during a certain number of independent (i.e. the event does not influence itself) 'trials', e.g. tossing a coin, or the outcome of emergency surgery. It is binomial because there are only *two* possible outcomes (heads or tails, survival or death). Given the probability of outcome A, the probability of outcome B is given by (1 − probability of outcome A).

A *Poisson* probability distribution describes the frequency with which a discrete random event occurring at a constant mean rate (e.g. atrial fibrillation, or mortality from a disease) is seen in a certain period. It is discrete because the event either occurs or does not occur. The probability of an individual event should be independent (e.g. one person's death does not influence the life-expectancy of another).

For the majority of medical research, which involves large numbers of observations, binomial and Poisson variables can be approximated by the normal distribution.

The **t-distribution** is derived from the normal distribution and is used for small sample sizes of a normally distributed variable (typically $n \leq 60$). The 'normality' of the variable is often assumed. As would be expected, the smaller the sample size the larger the SEs of its estimates of the population parameters. A **t-value** is similar in concept to a z-score and used in a similar way: both are measures of an estimate (e.g. population mean) or a difference (e.g. between two sample means) as a multiple of that estimate's or difference's SE.

There are various methods for calculating the SEs of statistics based on small samples, which depend on the particular statistic being calculated. The probabilities of the associated t-values, which are available in tables, are calculated using degrees of freedom (given by $n - 1$ for one sample and $n_1 + n_2 - 2$ for two samples).

SIGNIFICANCE TESTING

Much of medical research is about comparing two or more sets of data and determining whether they are different. **Significance** is a statistical concept used to determine whether the degree of difference between the data sets is sufficiently unlikely to have occurred by chance to suggest that they are in fact from different groups.

These scenarios are often stated as **hypotheses**. The **null hypothesis (H_0)** is that there is no difference between the groups (and therefore the data sets), while the **alternate hypothesis (H_1)** asserts that there is a difference. The analysis is usually conducted under the assumption that H_0 is correct, so that if a significant difference is found between the data sets H_0 is rejected in favour of H_1.

It is important before conducting a study to estimate how large it will have to be in order to manifest a significant difference in whatever measure the investigators have adopted. This will depend on the scale of the difference anticipated (sometimes called **effect size**); a large difference will be revealed by a relatively small study, whereas a small difference will require a large study to pick it up.

If a study is too small, there may be insufficient evidence to reject an incorrect null hypothesis, i.e. the study fails to reveal the genuine difference that exists between the groups. This is known as a **type II error**, and its probability is denoted by β. The probability of not committing a type II error is therefore given by $(1 - β)$ and is called the **power** of a test. This is the probability that the null hypothesis will be correctly rejected, i.e. that it is false and recognized as such.

β may be estimated from previous research, pilot studies, or set arbitrarily (often at 0.2, giving a power of 80 per cent). A power calculation estimates the number of subjects necessary to translate an effect size into a significant difference. In any paper that fails to reject H_0, a power calculation would help to rule out a type II error.

In order to decide whether a difference is sufficiently large to be deemed significant, we must first determine what range of values, for whatever statistic we are interested in (e.g. mean), might have been expected to occur by chance (i.e. the 'insignificant' range). This range depends on the degree of data dispersion.

For example, with a normally distributed variable, investigators may decide that a z-score outside 1.96 standard deviations of the mean ($P < 0.05$) is sufficiently unlikely to have occurred by chance for them to conclude that the groups from which the data were compiled are in fact different. This particular criterion is termed **significant at the 95 per cent level**, since they would have expected 95 per cent of values to lie within this range (because the probability of any normal variable being within 1.96 standard deviations of the mean is 0.95).

This range, within which the majority of values are expected to be (the exact proportion being determined by the level of significance), is called a **confidence interval**

(CI). The boundaries of this range are called **confidence limits.** A 90 per cent CI is the range within which 90 per cent of the values are expected to be (z-score within ± 1.645); a 95 per cent CI is the range within which 95 per cent of the values are expected to be (z-score within ± 1.96), and so on. A value lying outside these ranges is therefore regarded to be significant at the 90 per cent or 95 per cent level respectively. By convention, the 95 per cent significance level is commonly adopted.

In their results, researchers should use standard errors when estimating a parameter's CIs from a sample. For example, the 95 per cent confidence interval for the population mean is given by:

$$\text{CI (95 per cent) for } \mu = \text{from } (\bar{x} - 1.96 \times \text{SE}) \text{ to } (\bar{x} + 1.96 \times \text{SE})$$

The formulae for CIs of other values such as proportions and ORs are different, but in principle they all span the middle 95 per cent (or whatever significance level is chosen) of the distribution of that statistic.

A **type I error** is incorrectly rejecting the null hypothesis, i.e. wrongly concluding that there are group differences. If we set the significance level at 95 per cent, then we would expect to make this error 5 per cent of the time. Hence the probability of committing a type I error (denoted by α) is determined by the significance level.

In an effort to get a significant result, investigators may:

- extend the study beyond the original time-frame until some statistical difference is eventually manifest
- look for a significant difference between any two variables (data dredging), whether or not they are valid or provide any useful information
- relax the significance criteria
- change the outcome measure/use a surrogate measure instead of something more clinically relevant.
- ignore drop-outs: analysis should be carried out on an **intention to treat** basis. Subjects who drop out are regarded as failures (of whatever treatment-group they were recruited into) and included in the analysis as such. Where necessary, the last known measurement or result is 'carried forward' in order to plug any gaps in the final data set. If only participants who completed the study are considered, this is **completor analysis** and tends to over-emphasize the differences.

ONE AND TWO-TAILED TESTS

A one-tailed test considers the probability in one direction, i.e. above **or** below a particular z-score. A two-tailed test considers the probability in both directions, i.e. above **and** below the positive and negative values of a z-score. For example:

In a one-tailed test, $[P(z) < -1.645] = [P(z) > 1.645] = 0.05$ (95 per cent level significance)

In a two-tailed test, $[P(z) < -1.96] + [P(z) > 1.96)] = 0.05$ (95 per cent level significance).

Since it is often not known in which direction the population parameter lies with respect to the sample statistic, two-tailed tests are more common.

CHI-SQUARED TEST (χ^2)

This is used in comparing two or more categorical variables, e.g. housing status versus mental illness. Only the actual frequencies of observations can be used, not proportions or other derived statistics. The data is displayed in a table, such as in Table 18.3 (the figures used are for illustrative purposes only).

Table 18.3

	Affective illness			Schizophrenia		
	Observed (O)	Expected (E)	$(0 - E)^2/E$	Observed	Expected	$(0 - E)^2/E$
Homeless	19.00	24.33	1.17	32.00	26.67	1.06
Council	29.00	23.37	1.35	20.00	25.63	1.24
Renting	15.00	19.08	0.87	25.00	20.92	0.80
Ownership	20.00	16.22	0.88	14.00	17.78	0.80
Total	83.00	83.00	4.28	91.00	91.00	3.90

If we assume there is no difference between the housing status of the two groups, we would *expect* the proportions of people in the various housing categories to be the same for both groups; this is the null hypothesis, H_0. For example, under H_0 the proportion of those with affective illness who were homeless would be the same as the proportion of those with schizophrenia who were homeless, and so on down the rows.

The expected frequencies are calculated by first splitting the total observations in a particular row according to the ratio of the column totals. For example, the expected values for the homeless category are given by multiplying the total number of homeless (19 + 32) with the proportion of people with affective illness [83/(83 + 91)] and the proportion of people with schizophrenia [91/(83 + 91)], giving 24.33 and 26.67 respectively. This procedure is repeated to build up a column of expected frequencies. Note that the totals of the expected values equal those of the observed values across the rows as well as down the columns (e.g. in the last low, 20 + 14 = 16.22 + 17.78), which serves as a useful check for the calculations.

Essentially, we want to measure how different the observed and expected frequencies are. If there is a significant difference, we can say the proportions of observed frequencies in the two groups are not the same and that the null hypothesis is therefore wrong; there is in fact an inter-group difference in housing status. Note that we do not know in which direction the difference may lie, and so should carry out a two-tailed test.

The differences between the observed and expected values are squared (so they do not cancel each other), divided by the expected frequency and then added together to give a measure of the total degree of difference down the rows. This gives the results 4.28 and 3.90, which are then summed to give the overall χ^2 **statistic** 8.18. For a 2 × 2 table, a quicker formula for the χ^2 statistic is $[(ad - bc)^2 (a + b + c + d)]/[(a + b)(c + d)(b + d)(a + c)]$.

It turns out that χ^2 statistics are normally distributed and so their probabilities are available in tables. Consideration must be given to the degrees of freedom (d.f.), which in the case of a table is given by (rows − 1) × (columns − 1). Only the observed columns and labelled rows are included in this calculation, so that in the above example the d.f. is given by (4 − 1) × (2 − 1) = 3 (for a 2 × 2 table the d.f. = 1).

Looking up 8.18 at 3 d.f. in a χ^2 table, we see that the probability is 0.04. This is significant at the 95 per cent significance level (i.e. $P < 0.05$). Hence, we conclude that the null hypothesis is rejected at the 95 per cent significance level and that there is a difference in housing status between the two groups.

Note that at the 99 per cent level of significance, where we require $P < 0.01$, we would not reject H_0. However, we cannot by inference conclude that H_0 is correct. This illustrates the general principle that non-rejection of H_0 is not the same as saying it is accepted, only that there is insufficient evidence (at the stated level of significance) to disprove it.

DIFFERENCES BETWEEN MEANS

The mean of a sample, as an estimate of the population mean, has a SE. Therefore, the difference between two means will also have a SE. It turns out that if we took multiple samples from a population, the differences between the means of the samples follow the normal distribution. For large samples (say $n \geqslant 30$), we can assess the 'significance' of the difference (i.e. decide whether or not the samples are likely to be from the same population) in two ways.

The variance of the differences between two means is essentially the sum of their individual variances. So, the SE of the difference, SE(diff), is given by $\sqrt{[(s_1^2/n_1) + (s_2^2/n_2)]}$, and its 95 per cent CI ranges from $[(\bar{x}_1 - \bar{x}_2) - 1.96 \times \text{SE(diff)}]$ to $[(\bar{x}_1 - \bar{x}_2) + 1.96 \times \text{SE(diff)}]$, ignoring the sign of $(\bar{x}_1 - \bar{x}_2)$. If the difference lies within this range, it is not significant. Alternatively, we could calculate the z-score for the difference between the means, given by $(\bar{x}_1 - \bar{x}_2)/\text{SE(diff)}$, and look up its probability (i.e. P-value). Note that for paired data (e.g. case–control/cross-over studies) the methodology is different.

For small samples of normally distributed data, the t-test is used (see below).

ANOVA (an acronym for analysis of variance) compares the data of multiple groups to ascertain whether there is a significant difference between them. The **F ratio** is the degree of variation between group means relative to the variation within the groups. An F ratio >1 suggests the means are from different groups rather than from different samples of the same group.

SPECIFIC SIGNIFICANCE TESTS

- *Mann–Whitney U test*: a non-parametric test used to compare two sets of data. The U statistic is essentially a measure of where the values in the two sets appear relative to each other when they are all ranked together in ascending order. Under H_0, we would expect there to be no significant difference between the number of times a value in one set appears higher in the rankings than a value from the other. Once U is calculated it is compared against the probability distribution of U under H_0.
- *Wilcoxon rank-sum test*: the numerical differences (ignoring the sign) between the individual values of two sets of data are ranked, then the ranks of the positive and negative differences are summed separately. The lower of the two sums is called the T statistic, and under H_0 we would expect the T-statistic to be close to the mean of

these two values (as indeed we would the higher value). This test has been shown to be equivalent to the Mann–Whitney U test.

- *Student's* t-*test*: based on the *t*-distribution, this test is used to compare the means of two (small) sets of normally distributed data. The exact calculation varies according to whether the two sets are unpaired (independent samples) or paired (e.g. matched groups or two samples from the same group), and whether their variances are roughly equal. The probabilities of *t*-values can be looked up in a table at $(n_1 + n_2 - 2)$ d. f.
- *Kruskal–Wallis test*: this is a non-parametric one-way ANOVA.
- *Fisher's exact probability test*: this is used to compare small data sets of categorical variables (for large sets the χ^2 test may be used), typically 2×2 tables where the expected frequencies are <5. Because the data sets are small, it is not necessary to approximate using the χ^2 distribution; the exact probabilities can be calculated instead.
- *McNemar test*: obtains a *z*-score for the degree of difference between two sets of non-parametric (i.e. nominal or categorical) data, which can then be looked up in a normal distribution probability table.

CORRELATION

This is a measure of association; of how one variable changes in relation to another. For example, we might expect height and weight in children to be strongly correlated (i.e. as one changes, so does the other), but not their height and eye colour. The **strength** of correlation is denoted by the correlation coefficient, *r*.

r may be positive (the variables change in the same direction) or negative (they change in opposite directions). Note that the degree of change is less important than the consistency of change, i.e. two variables which always change together (one cannot be altered without producing a change in the other) will have a larger *r* than two variables which only sometimes change together, even if the latter involve more dramatic changes.

r may range from -1 (perfect negative correlation) to $+1$ (perfect positive correlation). A correlation coefficient of 0 suggests a complete absence of correlation. Extrapolating a correlation in order to 'fill-in gaps' or expand the range of the data is valid but entirely speculative. There is no guarantee the correlation persists beyond the available data, and extrapolation may encourage spurious conclusions.

Often, a scattergram of one variable plotted against another will allow a simple visual assessment of the degree and nature of any potential correlation; it may be possible to draw a **line of best fit** across the data. However, there are statistical methods for calculating *r* precisely.

For continuous data with an approximately linear relationship (this includes many variables encountered in medical literature), **Pearson's correlation coefficient** is an appropriate measure of association (also called the 'method of least squares' or 'linear regression'). The formula gives the ideal line of fit such that the total (vertical) difference between all the individual points and the line is as small as possible.

For non-parametric (e.g. categorical) data, **Spearman's rank correlation coefficient** may be used. This method involves assigning the data a rank order (both data sets must be ranked in the same direction, i.e. lowest to highest or vice versa), and then calculating the total degree of difference between the individual rankings (*not* the actual data). The correlation coefficient is expressed as r_s.

It is important to appreciate that correlation does not imply causation. Nor does it imply a direct relationship; the variables may both be related to some third factor rather than each other.

Multiple regression is used to establish how a variable alters in relation to more than one other variable, i.e. how a dependent variable changes with respect to two or more independent variables, or **predictors** (e.g. how weight correlates with height AND waist-size). We might also be interested in how any two of the variables are correlated with each other, ignoring the other variables. These sorts of analyses are usually done by computer and are called multivariate statistical tests.

SYSTEMATIC REVIEW/META-ANALYSIS

A systematic review is a complete survey of the research base in accordance with clear inclusion/exclusion criteria designed to address a clearly defined question. Publications should be assessed on their methodology and relevance, not their results. Essentially, the same ideas discussed above with regard to sampling apply, only with papers instead of people.

Because the overall 'population' of relevant papers is likely to be small, an effort should be made to look for and consider every one of them. This will include online databases, libraries, Index Medicus, contacting authors directly (sometimes for the raw data itself), looking up references and so on. The Cochrane Collaboration is a good example of systematic review.

A **funnel plot** can help gain perspective on the varying results likely to be seen among the studies identified in a systematic review. The effect sizes of individual studies are plotted against some measure of reliability (i.e. the likely 'repeatability' of the results). Suitable measures might be sample size, the SE of the results or the **precision** of the study (inversely related to the SE).

As might be expected, reliable studies tend to converge towards a particular effect size, with smaller studies giving results on either side of this value. This gives rise to the characteristic funnel-like (i.e. triangular) appearance of the plot. If there is a scarcity of data on one side of the funnel, this suggests a degree of **publication bias** (typically studies with negative results are published less often than those with positive results).

A **sensitivity analysis** assesses how 'fragile' (or robust, depending on your viewpoint) the conclusions of a review are, by considering how the results/conclusions would be affected by altering such factors as the inclusion/exclusion criteria, quality ratings (of individual studies) etc. If any such 'tampering' results in a different conclusion, the review is not definitive.

Meta-analysis is the pooling and interpretation of data collated by systematic review. The individual studies are **weighted** according to their estimated reliability (typically weight $= 1/SE^2$, though there is no fixed rule for assigning weight). In theory a meta-analysis carries greater authority because its conclusions are based on a larger data set than any of its constituent studies. The QUOROM statement is an international guideline on conducting meta-analyses.

The results of meta-analyses are often presented in a **forest plot** (or 'blobbogram'). The data are first collated or re-analysed to give confidence limits for the **same measure** of difference (e.g. relative risk) for each of the studies. These are then depicted as horizontal lines across a vertical **line of no difference** (e.g. RR = 1), giving an overall indication of where the evidence lies. The point estimate of the particular measure under consideration (i.e. the actual value whose confidence limits have been given) is marked as a square in the middle of each line, its size given by the weight assigned to that particular study.

The pooled data are usually represented as a diamond-shape at the bottom of the plot. Respectively, the height, width and position of the diamond represent the size of the data pool, the combined CI and where the pooled data sits with respect to the line of no difference. Once again, a diamond that crosses the line of difference does not mean the H_0 is accepted, only that there is (still) insufficient evidence to reject it at whatever level of significance the meta-analysis adopted.

A meta-analysis may be compromised by the degree of heterogeneity among its constituent studies (i.e. the more different the individual results, the harder it is to interpret their overall meaning). A measure of the heterogeneity (e.g. a χ^2 test) should therefore be included.

ECONOMIC ANALYSIS

These are efficiency studies designed to assess whether or not a particular course of action is 'worth it'. There are several ways to approach this question.

- *Cost-minimization analysis*: only the input costs are considered (typically money), with all other factors presumed to be equal, e.g. buying a product on special offer (such as '10 per cent off') which is on the supermarket shelf right next to the same product at full price. The products themselves, the consequences of buying the product and all other costs put into procuring the product are assumed to be identical.
- *Cost–benefit analysis*: all inputs and outputs are converted into money and added up, e.g. is it worth driving to a station selling petrol at 1p/L cheaper than one 2 miles closer? Clinical cost can be difficult to quantify in monetary terms.
- *Cost-effectiveness analysis*: costs of achieving a specific output or result (e.g. 2-year survival post-diagnosis of oesophageal cancer) by different means are compared. Allows a cost comparison of different treatments (e.g. conservative versus surgical) but cannot compare different outcomes (e.g. 2-year survival versus 5-year survival, or 2-year survival versus weight change).
- *Cost-utility analysis*: the output measure is a composite of quantitative and qualitative scores, e.g. quality-adjusted life years (QALYs). The subjective aspect of the qualitative component can be difficult to standardize. Allows comparisons between diverse interventions (providing the outcomes can all be converted into the same units). Takes **opportunity cost** into consideration, i.e. paying for one intervention means that alternatives cannot be afforded.

Costs may be described as **direct** (usually monetary: staff pay, drugs, investigations etc.) or **indirect** (non-monetary: convalescence, pain etc.). These terms are used inconsistently and it should be ascertained exactly what the authors mean by them.

A sensitivity analysis should be carried out to assess how altering the input costs might affect the results. A **one-way** analysis considers the effect of changing individual variables up or down. An **extreme** scenario is a form of one-way analysis in which individual variables are raised/lowered to their maximum/minimum. In a **probabilistic** analysis (Monte Carlo analysis) multiple variables are adjusted in plausible directions/amounts.

In appraising an economic analysis, particular attention should be paid to what the authors are attempting to compare and whether they have adopted a valid measure. Note that **efficacy** relates to theoretical (*in vitro*) results, and **effectiveness** to actual (*in vivo*) results. For example, is D_2-receptor occupancy necessarily a valid measure of antipsychotic effectiveness?

QUALITATIVE ANALYSIS

Perhaps more so than in any other type of research, common sense is the most useful tool in critically appraising a qualitative paper. The five questions raised at the beginning of this chapter remain a useful template, but there is no definitive guide on how to appraise such papers as they contain highly subjective information.

Qualitative research cannot be easily measured, rendering statistical analysis difficult. What is much more important is the methodology (how and what information was collected?) and validity (did the authors assess what they intended to and was this the right thing to have assessed?). The design should be described clearly and thoroughly, and at each step the reader should ask: *Why was this done/not done? Does this design adequately address the aims of the study, and what are its strengths/limitations?*

Any changes/adaptation made during the course of the study should be highlighted and explained. In particular, the authors need to have considered their relationship with the study and the subjects and what effect this relationship, and any changes they may have made, had on their results/conclusions. There is much greater scope for bias in qualitative research, both in sampling and in the gathering of information. However, there is a growing body of work on how to structure and implement the gathering of such information to minimize this potential pitfall.

Despite its apparent 'scientific' limitations, qualitative research is increasingly recognized as an important aspect of medical research, since few day-to-day questions about an individual patient's management can really be answered with a number. As is often said on ward rounds – 'don't treat the test result, treat the patient.'

EPIDEMIOLOGY

This is the study of disease distribution in a population. It is used in assessing aetiology (the cause of disease) and prognosis (the course of disease).

DESCRIBING DISEASE

- *Prevalence*: number of cases in a population at any point in time (point prevalence).

- *Prevalence rate (PR)*: prevalence divided by the number of people at risk. **Point PR**: data collected at one time; **Period PR**: data collected over a given period. PR approximates to incidence rate × average disease duration.
- *Incidence*: number of new cases arising in a given period.
- *Incidence rate*: incidence divided by the number of people at risk *or* length of time at risk.
- *Cumulative incidence rate*: incidence divided by the number of people at risk who are disease free.

COMPARING DISEASE

- *Relative risk*: risk of disease in exposed divided by risk of disease in unexposed, i.e. how many more times do exposed persons become diseased than non-exposed individuals?
- *Attributable risk (risk difference)*: difference in rate of occurrence (incidence) between exposed and non-exposed, i.e. how many new cases are due to the risk factor?
- *Attributable fraction*: attributable risk divided by total rate of occurrence in exposed population, i.e. what proportion of disease is due to the risk factor?
- *Population attributable risk*: the excess risk of disease posed by an exposure multiplied by the number exposed, i.e. how many cases in the population are due to the risk factor?

CAUSATION

A risk factor for a disease is one that increases the chances of contracting it, i.e. it contributes to the onset of the disease but is not directly causative:

Predisposing factors – create a susceptibility
Precipitating factors – closely associated with disease onset
Pathophysiological factors – mechanism by which a disease is expressed
Pathoplastic factors – influence the expression of disease
Perpetuating factors – maintain an established disease
Prognostic factors – influence disease outcome.

Many unifactorial disorders have an identified cause based on Koch's postulates (1882):

- the organism must be present in every case of the disease
- the organism must be isolated and grown
- the organism must be able to cause the disease when inoculated into susceptible host
- the organism must be recovered from that host and identified.

When such evidence is not available, or complex multifactorial systems are involved, Austin Bradford Hill's criteria may be used (1965):

- *Temporality*: the cause precedes the effect
- *Strength*: exposure vs. non-exposure produces significant difference in disease
- *Dose–response*: increased exposure produces increased effect
- *Reversibility*: reduction in exposure reduces disease occurrence

- *Consistency*: similar association has been found previously/since
- *Specificity*: one cause leads to one effect
- *Plausibility*: the association is concordant with current knowledge.

Table 18.4   Evidence of cause from studies

Study design	Additional evidence	Strength of hypothesis
Hypothesis alone	Plausibility	
Case report	Specificity	
Meta-analysis	Consistency	
Cross-sectional	Dose-response	
Case–control	Strength	
Cohort study	Temporality	
Clinical trial	Reversibility	Strongest

There is no gold-standard for deciding whether an association is causal. In assessing an association arising from a study (Table 18.4), consider whether the observed association could be due to:

- bias in selection or measurement
- confounding factors
- chance.

If not, then the null hypothesis of no difference can be rejected and a causal explanation for the association sought.

DIAGNOSIS

An ideal diagnostic test should be:

> Sensitive
> Specific
> Simple
> Safe
> Sound (i.e. reliable!)

For serious diseases, it is appropriate to have less stringent criteria/cut-off points (i.e. increased sensitivity), and so minimize false negatives (which will ↑ false positives). Highly stringent criteria (high specificity) will minimize false positives but ↑ false negatives.

PROGNOSIS AND TREATMENT

Prognostic factors are those that influence the course of an illness.

- *Natural history*: course of an illness without intervention
- *Clinical course*: course of an illness with medical intervention.

MEASURES OF OUTCOME

- Symptoms and signs: severity, response, remission, relapse
- Markers: diagnostic tests, social/physical functioning
- Diagnosis: recovery, relapse
- Mortality: survival.

Survival analysis: The time-to-death from the point of recruitment (zero-time). This can be plotted in a survival curve, indicating the cumulative probability of surviving each preceding time interval. Patients lost from a study are removed or censored.

Appendix 1

Theorists in the analytical psychiatry, social sciences and psychology

Author	Key association	Author	Key association
Abraham	Psychoanalyst	Kretschmer	Body-build
Adler	Individual psychology	Kubler-Ross	Death and dying
Allport	Humanistic psychology	Latance	Social impact theory
Bannister	Repertory grid	Lidz	Marital skew
Bateson	Double-bind	Lorenz	Imprinting
Berne	Transactional analysis	Maslow	Hierarchy of needs
Binet	Intellectual ability	McClelland	Achievement
Bion	Group therapy	Mechanic	Illness behaviour
Borgadus	Social distance scale	Meyer	Psychobiology
Bowlby	Loss	Milgram	Obedience
Broca	Expressive dysphasia	Mowrer	Drives
Cannon-Bard	Thalamic emotion theory	Osgood	Congruity theory
Cattel	Personality trait theory	Parkes	Bereavement
Ellis	Rational-emotive therapy	Parsons	Sick role
Erikson	Psychosocial development	Pavlov	Classical conditioning
Eysenck	Personality theory	Perls	Gestalt therapy
Festinger	Cognitive dissonance theory	Piaget	Cognitive development
Fiedler	Contingency theory	Pilowsky	Abnormal illness behaviour
Freud, A.	Defence mechanisms	Rank	Primal anxiety
Freud, S.	Psychoanalysis	Rogers	Self-theory
Fromm-Reichman	Schizophrenogenic mother	Rogers	Self-concept psychotherapy
Goffman	Institutionalization	Rotter	Locus of control
Heider	Balance theory	Schacter	Cognitive labelling
Horney	Holistic psychology	Seyle	General adaption syndrome
Hull	Drive-reduction theory	Sheldon	Body-types
James-Lange	Causal emotion theory	Skinner	Operant conditioning
Jung	Analytical psychology	Sullivan	Interpersonal theory
Kelly	Personal construct theory	Thorndike	Law of effect
Klein	Object relations	Wernicke	Receptive dysphasia
Kohlberg	Moral development	Winnicott	Object relations
Kohut	Self-psychology	Wolpe	Reciprocal inhibition

Appendix 2

Theorists in psychiatry, psychopathology and diagnosis

Author	Key association
Asher	Munchausen's syndrome
Bach-y-Ritta	Episodic dyscontrol syndrome
Barker	Hospital addiction syndrome
Beard	Neurasthenia
Bleuler	Schizophrenia
Cameron	Loosening of associations
Ganser	Vorbegehen
Goldstein	Concrete thinking
Gull	Anorexia nervosa
Hare	Pseudohallucination
Kadinsky	Pseudohallucination
Kahn	Anankastic personality
Kasanin	Schizoaffective disorder
Koch	Psychopathic inferiority
Kraepelin	Dementia praecox
Langfeldt	Schizophreniform psychosis
Leonard	Bipolar affective disorder
Meyer-Gross	Oneroid states
Miller	Accident neurosis
Moeli	Vorbeireden
Morgan	Non-fatal deliberate self-harm
Pinel	Manie sans delirie
Prichard	Moral insanity
Russel	Bulimia nervosa
Schneider	Schizophrenic formal thought disorder
Spitz	Anaclitic depression
Stromgen	Brief reactive psychosis

Appendix 3

Neuroendocrine findings in psychiatric disorders

Test	Depression	Schizophrenia	Eating disorder	Chronic alcohol dependency	OCD	Alzheimer's disease
HPA axis						
DST	Non-suppression (50%)	Suppression (90%)	Non-suppression (50%)	Non-suppression (25%)	Normal	Non-suppression (25%)
CRH challenge	Blunted ACTH	Normal	Blunted ACTH	Unknown	Normal	Blunted ACTH
CSF CRH	High (inconsistent)	Normal	High	Unknown	Unknown	Normal
HPT axis						
T_3/T_4	Normal	Normal	Low	Normal	Normal	Normal
TSH	Normal	Low (15%)	Normal	Normal	Normal	Normal
TRH challenge	Blunted (30%)	Normal	Blunted	Unknown	Unknown	Normal
	Augmented (15%)					
Thyroid autoantibodies	High (20%)	High (10%)	Normal	Unknown	Unknown	Normal
HPG axis						
Oestrogens	Normal	? Low	Low	Normal	Unknown	Unknown
LHRH challenge	Inconsistent	Unknown	Blunted	Unknown	Unknown	Unknown
Prolactin						
Serotonergic challenge	Blunted	Blunted	Unknown	Unknown	Blunted	Unknown
Growth hormone						
Basal	Blunted diurnal rhythm	Inconsistent	High	Normal	Blunted (30%)	Normal
Clonidine challenge	Blunted	Blunted (mild)	Unknown	Unknown	Blunted (30%)	Normal
Insulin challenge	Blunted	Unknown	Unknown	Normal	Blunted	Normal

Appendix 4

Cell membrane second messengers

	Hormones	Neurotransmitters	AA
Increases cAMP	ACTH, TSH, LH/FSH PTH, Calcitonin Glucagon G_2, Vasopressin V_2	Adrenergic β_1, β_2 5-HT$_4$, 5-HT$_6$, 5-HT$_7$ Dopamine D_1, D_5 Histamine H_2	
Decreases cAMP	Opioids Somatostatin	Adrenergic α_2 5-HT$_{1abd}$ Acetylcholine muscarinic receptor M_1, M_2 Dopamine D_2, D_3, D_4	
Calcium	LHRH, TRH Vasopressin V_1, Angiotensin	Histamine H_1	
Inositol kinase	Insulin Growth factors		
Ion channel		Acetylcholine nicotinic receptor 5-HT$_3$	GABA Glycine Glutamate

Appendix 5

Compendium of neuropsychological tests

Function	Test	Regional basis
Summary measures	Premorbid IQ (NART)	Global
	Wechsler verbal IQ	
	Wechsler non-verbal performance IQ	
	Mini-mental state examination	
Attention and working memory		Multimodal association areas
Articulatory loop	Phonological similarity effect	
	Word length effect	
	Forward digit span	
Visuospatial sketch pad	Forward block sequence span	
Central executive	Backward digit span	
	Backward block sequence span	
	Letter cancellation test	
Response times and psychomotor speed	Tower of London (subscale)	Basal ganglia
Executive functions		Frontal lobe
Planning	Tower of London	
	Verbal fluency	
	Motor sequencing	
	Trail-making test	
	Wisconsin card-sorting test	
Language	Boston naming test	Parietal lobe (dominant)
Visuospatial	Rey–Osterrieth figure	Parietal lobe (non-dominant)
Memory – explicit		Temporal lobe (medial)
Immediate free recall	Paired word recall	
Delayed recall	Prose passage recall	
Verbal	Wechsler, logical memory	
Visual	Wechsler, visual memory	
Memory – implicit		Basal ganglia
Recognition memory	Paired word recognition	

References and further reading

REFERENCE TEXTS

Puri B, Tyrer P. *Sciences Basic to Psychiatry* 2nd edn. Edinburgh: Churchill Livingstone, 1998.
Gelder M, Mayou R, Cowen P. *Shorter Oxford Textbook of Psychiatry*. Oxford: Oxford University Press, 2001.
Johnstone EC, Lawrie S, Freeman CPL, Owens DGC, Sharpe M. *Companion to Psychiatric Studies* 7th edn. London: Churchill Livingstone, 2004.

REVISION TEXTS

Select **one** text that suits your style and is comfortable to read. Then learn it!

Buckley P, Prewette D, Bird J, Harrison G. *Examination Notes in Psychiatry* 4th edn. London: Hodder Arnold, 2004.
Puri BK, Hall AD. *Revision Notes in Psychiatry* 2nd edn. London: Hodder Arnold, 2004.
Stern J, Phelan M, Wright P. *Core Psychiatry* 2nd edn. Oxford: Elsevier International, 2004.

ADDITIONAL TEXTS

Brown D, Pedder J, Bateman A. *Introduction to Psychotherapy* 3rd edn. London: Routledge, 2000.
Brown T, Wilkinson G (eds). *Critical Reviews in Psychiatry* 3rd edn. London: Gaskell (Royal College of Psychiatrists), 2005.
Cookson J, Taylor D, Katona C. *Use of Drugs in Psychiatry* 5th edn. London: Gaskell (Royal College of Psychiatrists), 2002.
Greenhalgh T. *How to Read a Paper* 2nd edn. London: BMJ Books, 2000.
Munafo M. *Psychology for the MRCPsych* 2nd edn. London: Hodder Arnold, 2002.
Sims A. *Symptoms in the Mind* 3rd edn. London: Bailliere Tindall, 2002.
Taylor D, Paton C, Kerwin R (eds). *The Bethlem and Maudsley Prescribing Guidelines* 7th edn. Oxford: Martin Dunitz, 2003 (new edition due 2005).
World Health Organization. *ICD-10*. Geneva: World Health Organization, 1992.
Lawrie SM, McIntosh AM, Rao S. *Critical Appraisal for Psychiatry*. London: Churchill Livingstone, 2000.

Note: For the MRCPsych Part II wider reading is advisable (e.g. mental health law and the various psychiatric sub-specialties). Always have the latest edition of the college syllabus to help plan your study.

Index

Note: Page numbers in **bold** refer to figures or tables